9-2-82
AUG 1 1 1982

THE PROCESS
OF CLINICAL
SUPERVISION

THE PROCESS OF CLINICAL SUPERVISION

by
Gordon M. Hart, Ph.D.
Professor of Counseling Psychology
Department of Counseling Psychology
Temple University
Philadelphia, Pennsylvania

UNIVERSITY PARK PRESS
Baltimore

UNIVERSITY PARK PRESS
International Publishers in Science, Medicine, and Education
300 North Charles Street
Baltimore, Maryland 21201

Typeset by Maryland Composition Company
Manufactured in the United States of America by The Maple Press
Company

Library of Congress Cataloging in Publication Data

Hart, Gordon M.
The process of clinical supervision.

Includes Index.
1. Mental health—Study and teaching—Supervision. 2. Mental health—Study and teaching
(Internship) I. Title. [DNLM: 1. Mental health
services—Organization. WM 30 H325p]
RA790.8.H37   616.89'007   81-16211
ISBN 0-8391-1700-0   AACR2

Contents

Preface

The increased interest in supervision over the last 5 years has led to a corresponding increase in books and articles on this most important part of training clinicians in the mental health field. The time seems appropriate to draw together the thinking and research in supervision from the areas of psychology, social work, and psychiatry in order to present the state-of-the-art and also to describe new formulations about how supervision can be used more effectively.

This work is divided into three sections, each encompassing several chapters. The first section, Introduction to Clinical Supervision, contains definitions and clarifications of the terms *supervision, consultation,* and *training,* and introduces and differentiates three models of supervision. The second section, Models of Clinical Supervision, contains three chapters each of which describes a different model of supervision including an annotated typescript of an actual supervision session and a description of many techniques such as role-playing, audiotaping and videotaping, and group work. Chapter 3 focuses on the Skill Development Model; Chapter 4 describes the Personal Growth Model; and Chapter 5 covers the Integration Model. The third section of the book, Practice of Clinical Supervision, contains a detailed description of the developmental stages of supervision. How to establish a comprehensive supervision program in terms of model, modality (individual, group, or peer), and temporal application (delayed, immediate, and live) is found in Chapter 7.

This volume will be of interest to theoreticians and practitioners and is designed to provide for the needs of both groups. The integration of previously published research is of value in establishing what we presently know about supervision and thus points the way to future research. Research is important not only in theory-building but also in guiding the practitioner's day-to-day work with supervisees. An important contribution of this book is the large amount of practical suggestions that can be used by supervisors working with psychiatrists, social workers, psychologists, psychiatric nurses, counselors or others either during their training or on-the-job. A further contribution is the emphasis on the development of the supervisory process over time and how a supervisor must be ready to adopt new models and techniques as the supervisee learns and then establishes new goals. One final contribution is the examination of the models of supervision, the modalities, and temporal applications of them in lieu of the developmental stage of the supervisee, which will be of interest to theoreticians and front-line supervisors.

Any author who focuses on some aspect of clinical expertise in the mental health field should uncover a bit more of the complexity of the field. Too often authors see this process as one of simplification, which does little to help practitioners or researchers. The process of clinical supervision is complex, and the complexity is just beginning to be understood. Indeed, a relationship exists between the guiding elements of the supervisor, the supervisee, and the context upon the supervisory process but the complexity of their relationship is only vaguely seen. The complexity of this relationship is compounded by the belief that supervision changes over time in an evolutionary manner that inextricably links supervision to the changes that occur in the relationship among the supervisor, supervisee, and context. This volume is one step in understanding the complex process of clinical supervision and of helping supervisors to carry out their part in supervision with greater understanding of what they can do to make the process more effective for their supervisees.

Acknowledgments

I would like to gratefully acknowledge the many people who provided me the intellectual assistance in understanding supervision better, the technical assistance in completing this volume, and the emotional support throughout the entire process. I owe a great deal to the many doctoral students who took Seminar in Supervision with me since my teaching of the course beginning in 1973. It is through my observation of their audiotapes and videotapes of supervision sessions plus their penetrating questions and creative thinking that has helped me most in my work. I also have found great joy in chairing the doctoral dissertations of Bill Liberi, Lynn Rosen, Walt Ciecko, and Brenda Byrne on supervision, which have served as the research arm of my interests. My colleagues deserve special thanks for their reading of the chapters and offering their invaluable perspectives. Dr. Jim Smith of Temple University. Dr. Howard Liddle, now director of the family therapy division of the Institute for Juvenile Research in Chicago, and Dr. Audrey Maslin of Hood College were not only reviewers and editors but also dear friends. I would particularly like to single out the hours of work contributed by my research assistant, Sandy Chierici who is not only thorough in obtaining articles from the library but who is also a competent clinician and future supervisor.

I would also like to thank my wife, Judy, who did all of the typing, provided the necessary emotional support throughout the entire project , and helped my three children Keith, Brian, and Beth to understand why this project was so important.

SECTION I

INTRODUCTION TO CLINICAL SUPERVISION

Chapter 1

An Overview
of the Field

3

INTRODUCTION

Supervision has been feared as a practice and, until recently, neglected as a field of study. Fear stems in part from the common view of the supervisor as one who judges workers' competence. Neglect is fostered by the belief that anyone who is a competent worker will be a competent supervisor. Supervision, as a field of study, is filled with myths, unclear definitions and distinctions, and untrained supervisors who operate with good intentions as their main resource. Yet, above the clamor and confusion, mental health workers (e.g., psychologists, psychiatrists, and social workers) rate their supervision as the most valuable aspect of their professional development. Apparently, supervisors are doing something right and even quite powerful despite their inability to describe clearly their goals, theoretical model, or outcomes. Supervision should be investigated in order to determine what makes such a maligned and taken-for-granted field have such a large impact.

The observations discussed in this text are based on several beliefs about the process of supervision, about supervisors, and about supervisees. These beliefs are based on a thorough review of the literature on supervision from the mental health areas of psychology, psychiatry, and social work plus personal observations of over 100 supervisees and dozens of supervisors during a ten-year period.

Beliefs about Supervision

Supervision is a complex undertaking that is, at times, as unfathomable as psychotherapy. Some authors have chosen to reduce this complex process by taking a microscopic view of supervisory behavior, and others provide a macroscopic perspective. The former allows researchers to conduct carefully controlled laboratory studies and reduce supervision to certain measureable elements. This leaves practicing supervisors with the knowledge of what to do; for example, to give corrective feedback, but not how, when, and with whom to do it. The macroscopic view of supervision shows the enormously rich and intense interactions that occur in supervision, which helps supervisors know how to go about supervision in general but not specifically what to do. An investigation of data from both sources is provided here.

Supervision varies to some extent from psychology to social work to psychiatry in terms of some specific skills that supervisees are to acquire, but the process by which these behaviors are acquired is quite similar in these fields. A thorough review of the mental health literature shows that three basic models of clinical supervision exist.

Ongoing supervision in any field goes through similar developmental stages that, although they overlap, are distinct. Descriptions of what supervisees want, what they expect, what they receive, and how they value it have led to conceptualizations of patterns that occur as supervision progresses.

An overriding assumption is that supervision is effective, although few studies have compared supervised clinicians with unsupervised clinicians. A notable exception is Biasco and Redfering's (1976) study in which clients of supervised clinicians reported significant gains over clients of unsupervised clinicians. It is assumed throughout this text that although having supervision may be more effective in promoting clinical expertise than not having supervision, the appropriate *application* of supervision determines the positive or negative outcomes of supervision.

Beliefs about Supervisors

A general belief about supervisors is that they all want their supervisees to become more proficient according to some criteria. This wish to bring about supervisee competence suggests a desire to use one's sources of interpersonal power to cause change in supervisees. Change implies a movement from one's present position to a position that is more professionally desirable. In this way, supervisors assess each supervisee's level of development and work in some way to increase that level. Unfortunately, many supervisors assess and implement strategies to produce change, and they evaluate in the most informal and ineffective ways. Supervisors generally have constructive intentions, but often their implementations seem to fail.

Generally, the uneven performance of supervisors in all mental health professions is attributable to their lack of training in supervision, a work setting that does not promote the effective delivery of clinical supervision, and a profession that only recently has turned to the careful study of the processes and outcomes of supervision.

At another level, a stereotype exists among many clinicians that their supervisor has attained that position by virtue of some clinical expertise that far exceeds the expertise acquired by others, and that such expertise is directly related to or, indeed, synonymous with expertise in supervision. Many people have learned that a competent practioner is not necessarily a competent teacher; yet, the stereotype persists among both supervisees and supervisors themselves.

A further belief about supervisors is that they underestimate the difficulty of the change process implied in supervision. For some reason clinicians generally anticipate client or patient resistance to change in the counseling or psychotherapy process, but in supervision such anticipation does not seem to appear. It is assumed throughout this text that the supervision process is similar to other change processes such as teaching, psychotherapy, or child raising, and that resistances inevitably emerge.

A final belief is that a supervisor's effectiveness hinges more on the issue of evaluation than on any other issue. Not only are the end-of-term or annual evaluations important, but also evaluations that are done by the supervisor during every supervision session with every supervisee are critical to the outcome of the supervisory process. Some supervisors objectify and thus clarify the evaluation aspect of supervision through the use of rating scales or other such instruments. Other supervisors are sensitive to supervisees' fears of being negatively evaluated. Still other supervisors attempt to avoid the issue of evaluation by letting formal evaluations be done by another person such as an administrator which, of course, does not address the in-session evaluation that remains.

Of course, some supervisees may enter supervision with an exaggerated fear of the supervisor's evaluation, but this fear then becomes the beginning issue on which supervisor and supervisee focus. Furthermore, the supervisee's perception of his or her own competence may be the issue that needs attention, and excessive evaluation apprehension is an index of an unreasonably high criterion for competence and an excessive interest in attaining that criterion.

Beliefs about Supervisees

All supervisees in mental health professions have questions about their performance in both an absolute and a relative sense. In an absolute sense they want to know what behaviors are *most* effective with clients. They ask, "Should I be more confrontive with Charlie about his aggressive behavior?" or "What's the best agency in the city for handling a referral for Susan?" A belief that it is possible to identify *the most* effective strategy is probably naive, but practitioners ought to know if they are using *one of the most* effective strategies.

In a relative sense, mental health workers want to know how their performance compares to the performance of other workers who are similar in training, experience, or job assignment. They think, "How do I handle groups compared to other students you're supervising?" or "Do you think I'm as skilled in testing as Stan who came to the agency when I did?" Similarly, people want to know if their competence is increasing with time. They wonder, "Have my reports seemed better now than before?" or "Do you think I've been able to handle myself better with parents?" According to Mueller and Kell (1972), the need to know about one's competence is the single most important issue to be addressed during supervision.

A second belief about beginning mental health workers is that they want and need to know the professional roles that are expected of them. The professionalization or acculturation of new persons into a particular occupation means that certain expectations about behavior—roles, ethical responsibilities—are transmitted in a formal and informal manner. Those who learn how a professional mental health worker acts toward clients and colleagues rapidly feel comfortable and accepted. Some professionalization is accomplished through incidental learning and modeling by faculty or staff. Supervision can be used to help students or new staff members learn the appropriate professional roles and procedures in a more systematic manner.

A third belief regarding supervisees is that those people who have positive interactions in supervision will function more positively in their work. In a recent study of social workers, those who were satisfied with their supervision were also more satisfied with their work and had "better individual performance, less absenteeism, better agency performance and higher agency competence" (Olmstead & Christensen, 1973, p. 304).

In line with these beliefs, the purposes of this volume are to define supervision in terms that clearly differentiate supervision from other processes, to describe the goals and characteristics of three models of supervision, and to show supervisors how to apply these models within the developmental process of supervision. Each section of this book is devoted to one of these three purposes. In Chapter 1, supervision is described in terms of functions and how these functions are viewed throughout the various mental health professions. These functions yield the differentiation between administrative or managerial supervision and clinical supervision. Next, supervision is contrasted with training, consultation, and therapy in order to establish precise definitions of these terms.

BACKGROUND

Supervision in the mental health fields of psychiatry, social work, and psychology has developed independently thus making comparisons across fields difficult. One issue on which differences exist is the level of training of the supervisee. Level of training refers primarily to whether the supervisee is a student in training or a worker on the job. Reviews of supervision in psychiatry (Kagan & Werner, 1977) and in medicine (Kutzik, 1977) show that supervision takes place only during the training period and is replaced by consultation when the physician is on the job. Brammer and Wassmer (1977) reviewed supervision conducted in university psychology departments even though some supervision was done on-the-job with psychologists. Supervision in social work (called field instruction) is conducted during the formal training period and is continued in some form when the social worker takes a job upon completion of formal training (Kadushin, 1976; Kutzik, 1977; Vargus, 1977).

In all fields it is assumed that supervisees change as a result of their experiences and the demand characteristics of the context (training program or agency) in which they function. Because the experiences and contexts are different for students and beginning clinicians, supervision in training programs and agencies should be researched to determine what differences exist. In the field of social work Kadushin (1976) refers only to the supervision of workers, not students, but throughout his text he refers interchangeably to research done on students and workers, which suggests that his definition fits both groups. Vargus (1977), relying on the earlier survey research of Pettes (1967) and others in social work, suggested that differences exist between a university supervisor and an agency supervisor in terms of "what is taught, perceptions of students, and expectations of students; but it is more a degree of difference rather than an alternative supervisory process." With this point in mind, supervision is viewed in this text as a flexible process that can be applied both to students in training and clinicians in agencies. Future research, however, may delineate areas of significant differences.

A second issue concerning supervision across mental health fields is the lack of agreement about supervision as differentiated from training and consultation. The historical development of supervision described here may begin to show the differences and similarities among these terms. Of particular importance is the examination by Kutzik (1977) of supervision and consultation in both medicine and social work. Many of his observations and conclusions are applicable to supervision in psychology.

According to Kutzik, supervision existed in medicine since the 13th century in England where physicians supervised the work of other persons in medically-related occupations. As required training increased in these occupations, independence and competence of practioners increased. This trend led to an increase in supervision where physicians directly reviewed the work of untrained assistants and an increase in consultation where physicians met periodically with independently practicing paraprofessionals. Apothecaries, for example, treated many patients independently, consulting with a physician only on those cases that required assistance. Much later in the 1800s, in the United States, physicians hired and directly supervised surgical assistants, thus forming the base of modern medical supervision.

Currently, the supervision process of the medical profession takes place during the internship and residency years of a physician's training. The assumption is that following graduation, a physician/psychiatrist is now able to function as a fully independent clinician who does not need supervision but who may seek consultation when he or she deems it necessary or desirable. The fields of counseling and clinical psychology have adopted the same assumption; that is, psychologists who have received their doctorate do not need supervision but occasionally may need to consult with a colleague.

Supervised clinical experiences for psychologists in training did not become widely accepted until the last two decades—much later than it did in the psychiatric and social work fields. One impetus for strengthening supervision of psychologists was the passage of the Mental Health Act of 1963, which led to community mental health centers and, consequently, to the intermingling of professions under one roof (Kaslow, 1977). Psychologists not only developed a strong system for supervising students in training but also have provided empirical studies of supervision (Leddick & Bernard, 1980).

Supervision in social work, at least administrative supervision, began during the development of the charity organization societies and settlement houses of the late 1870s and 1880s. An educational component was not added to the administrative function until after 1900 (Kadushin, 1976). Apparently, the settlement houses used consultation, but public welfare relied on supervision. From the 1930s to the present, social work supervision could be either consultation (Kutzik, 1977) or a special type of supervision that is similar to consultation. Clearly, supervision in social work has evolved to a point where more highly trained and more experienced workers engage in consultation and less experienced and less trained workers receive some form of supervision. Supervision is practiced on-the-job more often in social work than in psychiatry or psychology.

Throughout this text, supervision is considered in terms of both students in training programs from paraprofessional to post-doctorate as well as those clinicians who have begun professional work and are being supervised in agency settings. Supervision is used commonly with students but is often changed or substituted for consultation when clinicians enter agency employment. Lack of precise use and application of terms such as supervision, training, and consultation has made research and theory building across fields more difficult.

DEFINITIONS

The goal of this section is to define relevant terms such as education, training, consultation, and supervision and to distinguish between administrative/managerial and clinical supervision. This will prepare the reader for the indepth comparison of training, consultation, and supervision in the following section.

Authors in all mental health fields have attempted to define supervision. Authors from psychiatry (Ekstein & Wallerstein, 1958, 1972; Fleming & Benedek, 1966; Schuster, Sandt, & Thaler, 1972), from psychology (Kell & Mueller, 1966; Mueller & Kell, 1972), and from education (Goldhammer, 1969) have described at length their methods of conducting supervision. Broader works by Hendrickson and Krause (1972), Kaslow (1977), and Kurpius, Baker, and Thomas (1977) survey the mental health field as a whole; only a few authors have written conceptual works on models of supervision (Boyd, 1978; Kurpius & Baker, 1977; Oratio, 1977).

Throughout this volume *education* is used generically—it refers to all forms of formal and informal learning of which training, supervision, and consultation are particular types. *Training* refers to formal educational experiences, usually conducted in a classroom format, in which specific knowledge and skills have been selected on an a priori basis by program (university or agency) administrators to be presented to students or employees. Training is a particular aspect of one's education that is designed to help all trainees meet certain standards established by a profession.

Supervision is also a formal educational experience but is a specific type of experience that is an important part of any comprehensive training program. Typically, supervision has been described by lists of functions or tasks that should be implemented (DeBell, 1963). Kurpius and Baker (1977) stated, "Supervision is the conceptualization, implementation, control, and management of training in applied circumstances and conditions" (p. 224). This definition is helpful as a starting point, but some description of the relationship between the supervisor and the supervisee is also needed. Brammer and Wassmer (1977) stated, "Supervision is the assignment of an experienced person to help a beginning student to learn counseling through the use of the student's own case material" (p. 44). Kutzik (1977) described the process in more detail. He defined supervision as "a continuous relationship of an organizational superior and subordinate—supervisor and supervisee, respectively—in which the latter is required to report regularly to the former on the state of his or her work and the supervisor provides direction that the supervisee is bound to follow" (p. 5).

The definition of supervision used in this volume combines the process partly described by Kutzik (1977), and the goal, partly described by Brammer and Wassmer (1977). For this volume, clinical supervision is an ongoing educational process in which one person in the role of supervisor helps another person in the role of the supervisee acquire appropriate professional behavior through an examination of the supervisee's professional activities. The important elements are that: 1) there is an ongoing relationship between supervisor and supervisee, 2) the supervisor does not have to be an organizational supervisor of the supervisee (as, for example, in peer supervision) although the roles of supervisor and supervisee are clear, 3) the content of the sessions may include a wide range of knowledge and skills that pertain to effective professional behavior with clients and colleagues, and 4) the focus is on the behavior of the supervisee as it occurs in present interpersonal interactions.

Consultation is an informal educational experience usually used in place of supervision. Kutzik (1977) described consultation as "a time-limited relationship of professional peers in which the consultee voluntarily seeks the advice of the consultant regarding a specific case or problem and decides whether or not to take this advice." His definition is based on typical practice in medicine, social work (Austin, 1960; Kutzik, 1972; Pettes, 1967; Rapoport, 1954), and community mental health in general (Caplan, 1970). Kurpius and Robinson (1978) concurred that, "many writers view the consultant as a collaborator who forms egalitarian relationships with the consultees to bring about change. In this collegial relationship, there is a joint diagnosis with emphasis on the consultees finding their own solution to their problems. The consultant serves as a catalyst or facilitator for the problem-solving process" (p. 322). Consultation differs from supervision in the roles of the participants and the length of time the processes are implemented.

In bureaucratic organizations such as universities and mental health agencies, administrators must oversee, direct, and evaluate the work of clinicians whether they are students or staff. This process has been termed *administrative* or *managerial* supervision (Black, 1975; Wiles & Lovell, 1975). The university professor or agency director, during *administrative* supervision, assists students or workers in following institutional procedures that help the organization function more effectively and efficiently. Such procedures would include attendance at meetings, keeping case records up to date and providing information on clients to other agency personnel. In contrast, *clinical* supervision focuses on the work of student or staff members in relation to clients or colleagues and includes areas such as assessment, diagnosis, counseling/psychotherapy, and referral. The distinction between these two terms is based on the purpose and the content of the supervision sessions. Administrative supervision is aimed at helping the supervisee as a part of an organization, and clinical supervision focuses on the development of the supervisee specifically as an interpersonally effective clinician. The content of administrative supervision centers on the effective performance of duties that directly benefit the organization, and clinical supervision examines the supervisee's performance of specific clinical tasks that affect the recipients of the service.

This distinction between administrative and clinical supervision is important because the focus of the entire volume is on clinical supervision not administrative supervision. Of course, many supervisors conduct both types of supervision, but these supervisors must clearly understand the differences between them in order to be effective at both.

For supervisors who conduct both administrative and clinical supervision, the issue of potential conflict has long been raised (Austin, 1956, 1960, 1961). Some authors in social work (Devis, 1965; Hanlan, 1972; Schwartz & Sample, 1972) strongly believe that these types of supervision should be separated. Representatives of psychiatry (Spiegel & Grunebaum, 1977) and of psychology (Arbuckle, 1963) also support a clear separation of roles. The assumption is that administrative supervision is tied to promotion, pay increases, etc., and so is inherently more evaluative than clinical supervision, which does not pertain as directly to such rewards and punishments. In this situation, supervisees will be anxious and therefore will react in various ways such as rebellion or ingratiation in order to avoid a negative report by their supervisor.

Kadushin (1976), referring to social workers, stated an opposite opinion: "There is no substantial empirical evidence that learning seriously suffers as a result, nor is there any good evidence that learning substantially improves when the educator is absolved of the responsibility for evaluating and grading" (p. 447). Kadushin used the work of Cruser (1958), Kledarias (1971), Olyan (1972), and his own study (Kadushin, 1973) to conclude that "although the literature of social work supervision continues to debate the problem, it [evaluation] does not seem to be much of a problem for supervisors" (p. 447).

A different perspective on this issue is taken in psychology by Mueller and Kell (1972) who believe that evaluation is always being conducted by a supervisor regardless of the type of supervision (administrative or clinical). A supervisee's behavior as evaluated in administrative supervision may be linked to career advancement; however, a supervisee's behavior as evaluated in clinical supervision involves one's sense of competence—an important part of one's interpersonal need structure. Therefore, it is assumed here that evaluation apprehension in supervisees is inevitable. Even when no formal administrative power is held by the supervisor, evaluation is the key issue that must be resolved by the supervisor and supervisee before progress can be made toward the goals of supervision. Instead of attempting to reduce anxiety by separating the administrative and supervisory roles, Mueller and Kell offered suggestions on how supervisors can address the evaluation issue in supervision sessions regardless of the structural or organizational circumstances that bring about the issue. Evaluation is one of the most important issues needing examination within clinical supervision.

The following section further clarifies the most frequently confused terms—training, consultation, and supervision. The lack of precise definitions and usage has led to uninterpretable research and inapplicable theories. With this clarification, theorists and practioners will be able to conduct their work more precisely. In addition, the two dimensions used here to differentiate supervision, consultation, and training are used later to differentiate the three models of supervision described extensively in this text.

DISTINCTIONS BETWEEN
TRAINING, SUPERVISION, AND CONSULTATION

A thorough review of the definitions and descriptions of supervision in psychology, social work, psychiatry, and education shows that there is confusion regarding the terms training, supervision, and consultation. Kutzik (1977) stated that "both professions, medicine, and social work, have used supervision and consultation throughout their histories, that both have at times confused one with the other—and with the training of students and neophytes" (p. 57).

Two factors differentiate training, supervision, and consultation: the amount of participation by the learner and the sources of power used to promote learning.

Participation by the Learner

The amount of participation by the learner refers to the extent that the learner chooses the goal to be accomplished, determines the material to be discussed or presented, and evaluates the results of the learning. In training, the goal and material to be presented are determined typically by faculty members or agency administrators. Usually, a common level of learning is assumed, and trainees are expected to attain a predetermined level of learning. Evaluation is conducted by a formal or informal assessment of the trainees' understanding of the material and occasionally of the effects of the process on the trainees' behavior. The purpose of evaluation is to help faculty members or agency administrators determine the effects of the training experiences.

In supervision, goals are largely determined by the supervisor with some input from the supervisee. Evaluation of supervision is usually conducted with some participation by the supervisee by means of mutual assessment of the supervisee's progress by the supervisor and supervisee. Overall, more active participation in goal setting, material to be discussed, and evaluation occurs in supervision than in training.

More active participation and individualization occurs in consultation than in supervision or training because the responsibility for identifying the goal lies solely with the consultee. Once the consultation process has begun, some cooperation may occur regarding material to be discussed but generally the consultee chooses the material to be examined. Finally, evaluation is left entirely to the consultee. The consultant may request feedback regarding the effects of the consultation process, although the consultee has no obligation to report the effects, which is in sharp contrast to training and supervision.

Sources of Power Used to Promote Learning

Every trainer, consultant, or supervisor tries to influence the trainee, consultee, or supervisee. The influencing process can be analyzed based on the type and amount of interpersonal power used by the trainer, supervisor, or consultant.

French and Raven (1960) categorized sources of power as being reward power, coercive power, positional power, expert power, and referent power. When examining training, supervision, and consultation according to these sources of power, certain distinctions emerge.

A trainer is usually an organizational superior to a trainee and possesses positional power over the trainee. The trainer's decisions and opinions can affect the trainees progress in the organization. Closely related is the trainer's power to praise, to grant time off, or to dispense positive recommendations to trainees (reward power) as well as punishment, failure, demotions, and discharge (coercive power).

Supervisors, like trainers, are usually organizational superiors (e.g., faculty, agency administrators) to their supervisees and so possess positional, reward, and coercive power. In consultation, however, a consultee has the option to choose a consultant who may or may not be an organizational superior. If a peer is chosen, then this consultant will have no positional power and less reward and coercive power than in training or supervision. Furthermore, in supervision and training the supervisees or trainees are expected to implement the suggestions or teachings delivered to them. In consultation, on the other hand, the opinion of the consultant may be disregarded by the consultee. No obligation exists on the part of the consultee to use the opinion or to report to the consultant on whether the opinion was used. Positional, reward, or coercive power are much more in evidence in training and supervision than in consultation.

The influencing process can also be based on other sources of power, namely, expert power and referent power. Expert power is derived from the degree of professional competence one has, and referent power is based on the strong positive feelings one person has for another. Kadushin (1976) combined positional, reward, and coercive power and called the category "formal" power (p. 98). He then placed referent and expert power into a category called "functional" power. Formal power is typically emphasized by supervisors in business and industry (Black, 1975) and functional power is usually practiced by supervisors in social service occupations.

A wealth of research has been conducted on sources of power and how they have been perceived by supervisees. Social workers surveyed by Olmstead and Christensen (1973) stated that expert power was the most important source of power in their position.

Kadushin (1974) also found that both Masters of Social Work supervisors and their supervisees view expert power as the main source of power. Psychological research by Hester, Weitz, Anchor, and Roback (1976) confirmed that counselors were attracted to their supervisors more because of perceived skillfulness of the supervisor than the counselors' perceived similarity of attitudes between themselves and the supervisor. Gale (1976) was surprised to find that 10 out of 61 psychiatric residents rated the teaching of their supervisors as good even though they rated rapport with the supervisor as poor. He concluded that the effects of a competent clinical supervisor were different from the effects of a personal relationship between supervisor and supervisee.

An important point is that expert power is based on the expertise of the consultant, trainer, or supervisor as *perceived* by the consultee, trainee, or supervisee. When supervisees, trainees, or consultees perceive a supervisor, trainer, or consultant as being more expert than they, expert power is present. Expertise may be inferred from a person's academic training and degrees, types of experiences, amount of experience, honors gained within the professional community, or other achievements, but actual expertise may never be determined. The greater the difference in perceived expertise among participants, the greater the expert power in training, supervision, and consultation. In consultation a person may seek a consultant who is similar in level of training and organizational position; however, once a person asks for consultation, the consultant is perceived to be at least minimally more expert than the consultee on the issue under consideration. This establishes what Haley (1963) termed a complimentary relationship in which each person plays roles that interact in a cooperative or agreeable fashion. Overall, expert power is a primary source of power in training, supervision, and consultation.

Identification of the supervisee with the supervisor (forming referent power) has been discussed at length in the psychiatric literature. Some authors such as Benedek (1954) have cautioned supervisors to avoid fostering strong identification by their supervisees. Others such as Tarachow (1963) and Grotjahn (1955) believe that identification with a supervisor is important and should be encouraged. Cohen and DeBetz (1977) thoroughly reviewed the psychiatric literature on this point and suggested that "a prevailing belief seems to be that the supervisor should offer himself as a transference figure for student identification." The degree of identification, however, is extremely important. If identification is so strong as to encourage a dependent mimicking of the supervisor, then such an identification is counterproductive. On the other hand, some identification is necessary because the first stage of supervision often consists of "imitative learning" (Fleming, 1953), which is highly desired by psychiatric residents (Chessick, 1971). For example, in a survey of 15 practicing psychiatrists, Schowalter and Pruett (1975) found that "the most useful trait most commonly mentioned by the graduates was that of the supervisor's sharing his style of work with the supervisee" (p. 709). The need for the demonstration of skills by the supervisor is apparently based on psychiatric residents' lack of specific skills training prior to supervision (Gardner, 1953) and to the high anxiety experienced by residents at the beginning of their residency (Spiegel & Grunebaum, 1977). Students in other professional areas have similar experiences (Balsam & Balsam, 1974) that encourage an identification with their supervisor. Identification is a powerful factor in establishing referent power.

Many issues arise from the dimensions chosen to differentiate training, supervision, and consultation. For example, what is the optimum level of participation among learners? What different goals should be accomplished via each process of training, supervision, and consultation? What are the effects of different sources of power when used to promote learning in the processes considered here? These issues are particularly important in supervision because of the emphasis consistently placed on them by supervisees (Gardner, 1953; Scott, 1969; Aiken, Smits, & Lollar, 1972; Kadushin, 1973). Furthermore, the use of these sources of power in supervision is an important determinant of the particular model of supervision one implements.

In the next section, the functions of supervision are described so that the intent of supervision, according to supervisors, is clarified. How these functions may be carried out is then described in Chapters 2 through 5 in terms of three models of supervision.

FUNCTIONS OF SUPERVISION

Functions of supervision include both products and processes. Products are the desired outcomes of supervision and processes are the techniques used to achieve the products. The desired outcomes or goals of clinical supervision are examined in this section, leaving the processes to be considered in detail in Chapter 2. With some conceptualization of the goals to be achieved by supervision, the models for achieving them can be constructed with greater clarity.

In his definitive text on supervision in social work, Kadushin (1976) stated that the principal functions of supervisors are administrative, supportive, and educative. As conceptualized in the previous section of this volume, supervision can be administrative and/or clinical. In Kadushin's terms, an administrative supervisor should carry out an administrative function; a clinical supervisor should carry out an educative function; and both types of supervisors should carry out a supportive function. The administrative function is briefly noted here to show the contrast between administrative and educational functions. The supportive function is mentioned only briefly here because it is examined later in more detail.

Administrative Function

The supervisor as administrator in a social service agency is responsible for directing and evaluating the work of supervisees in order to help the agency deliver services in the most effective and efficient manner possible. Decisions need to be made that increase the amount and/or quality of effective service delivered. Such decisions may place a supervisor in a wholly managerial position that undermines educative and supportive functions. As the term "middle-manager" suggests, supervisors are between upper-level administrators and staff who work directly with clients; consequently, supervisors have an administrative as well as a clinical function.

Furthermore, the goals of the agency require that individual staff members relinquish some of their idiosyncratic and autonomous behavior thereby conforming to a prescribed norm of behavior. When a supervisor interprets the goals of the organization and issues directives that demand conformity, relationships with supervisees built on enhancement of personal autonomy will suffer. Professionals, particularly in medicine and in psychiatry, have long described the need for practioners to strive for independent and autonomous control of their activities. The dynamic tension between organizational goals that promote conformity and worker goals centered on autonomy is a contextual factor that affects a supervisor's approach to supervisees.

Supportive Function

The supportive function is determined by the quality of the emotional relationship between supervisor and supervisee that has been viewed by some researchers as the most important component of effective clinical supervision. This function is implemented through "reassurance, encouragement, and recognition of achievement, realistically based expressions of confidence, approval and commendation, catharsis-ventilation, desensitization and universilization, and attentive listening which communicates interest and concern" (Kadushin, 1976). These procedures are similar to the facilitative conditions (Carkhuff, 1969) for all effective interpersonal relations. Regardless of administrative or clinical supervision—administrative or educational functions—a supportive relationship between supervisor and supervisee will promote the desired goals of the supervision process.

To consider the supportive aspect as a separate function is to imply that supervisors engage in supportive activities only at certain times, for example, when the supervisee displays stress related to the job. A different view is for support to be a base that undergirds both administrative and educative functions. In this way supervisors should be supportive of supervisees not only in times of stress but also at other times. Consequently, support will be viewed as a foundation that is necessary but not sufficient for maximally effective administrative or clinical supervision to occur.

Educative Function

The educative function of supervision is emphasized throughout the literature of the mental health professions and in business and industry. It is clear that supervision during a training program will have a large, if not exclusively, educational function; however, what educative role should the agency adopt? Watson (1973) stated that social workers should learn "social work philosophy and the history and policy of the agency; social work knowledge, techniques, and skills; self-awareness; available resources in the agency and the community; and the priorities of case service and the management of time" (p. 81).

In contrast to this broad statement by Watson, a review of the literature reveals four goals of the educative function:

1. Knowledge of the approaches deemed appropriate and used by the professionals in a particular agency or field
2. Clinical knowledge and skills that were established at a rudimentary level during formal training
3. Conceptualization of client behavior
4. Self-awareness

These goals are the basic goals that models of supervision have been designed to accomplish with beginning supervisees. Other goals will be more important to supervisees once they have attained these fundamental goals (Cleghorn & Levin, 1973).

Knowledge of Professional Roles   Professional roles refer to the methods by which a newly-trained worker can deliver service according to the norms of professional behavior. Just as socially appropriate behavior exists, so does professionally appropriate behavior (Strauss, 1964). As Kadushin (1976) stated, "Educational supervision is the context for role transition from lay person to professional, providing the supervisee with his sense of occupational identity" (p. 129). This area of education for beginning workers is essential if they are to establish a strong professional identity and a cohesive relationship with their agency colleagues. Furthermore, a worker who is new to an agency (even someone with years of experience elsewhere) needs to learn the accepted means for delivering service in this new setting.

Clinical Knowledge and Skills   The second goal of the educative function of supervisors is to increase the clinical knowledge and skills that began during formal training. Such clinical skills include establishing relationships, making diagnostic judgments, delivering effective treatment through individual, group, or family psychotherapy, evaluating client progress, making referrals, termination, and conducting follow-up procedures. Supervisors in formal training programs begin with basic skills and work to the level of skills that the ability of the supervisee and the length of the program will allow. Many supervisors believe that a high level of skills is an unrealistic goal during formal training because practical experience of the students is often limited. Consequently, several years in active professional service under supervision are believed to be necessary for the attainment of high level skills. This view is strongly held by social workers, less so by psychologists, and least by psychiatrists, as indicated by the use of supervision by these groups. That is, social workers use supervision extensively for new workers, psychologists use supervision less, and psychiatrists use it very little. It seems apparent that through supervision, workers' skills can be enhanced and refined in a thorough and comprehensive manner.

Case Conceptualization   A third objective of the educative function of supervision is to develop a supervisee's conceptualization of the social, cultural, and behavioral patterns of clients (individuals, groups, or organizations). Psychiatry (Kagan & Werner, 1977) placed a strong emphasis on case conceptualization among supervisees in training programs. Yet, during formal training a student can encounter only a limited number of cases in which to learn principles of client behavior. This goal of supervision suggests that a supervisee (student or worker) devote time in supervision to analyzing information about clients and their backgrounds, comparing present clients with past clients, and generating hypotheses on which treatment strategies can be based. The accumulation of experience takes time; yet, the discussion of these experiences in supervision can aid in the assimilation of experiences by students and workers (Goin & Kline, 1974).

Self-Awareness   Self-awareness by the supervisee refers to *insight*, which is defined as knowledge and understanding of one's own interpersonal behavior including motives plus affective sensitivity, which is defined as knowledge of one's own feelings as they are experienced in interpersonal situations. Vargus (1977) and Kadushin (1976) concur that in social work, "The supervisor has the responsibility of teaching the worker about himself as well as teaching the worker about people, problems, places, and process" (Kadushin, 1976, p. 155). From the viewpoint of psychology, Patterson (1964) stated, "It [supervision] is concerned with the development of sensitivity in the student, of understanding and ability to communicate that understanding, of therapeutic attitudes, rather than techniques, specific responses, diagnostic labeling, or even identifying or naming presumed personality dynamics in the client" (p. 48).

Supervisors in psychology, social work, and psychiatry generally agree on the value of personal awareness as a goal of supervision; however, their definitions of personal awareness vary greatly. For some supervisors self-awareness means insight and/or affective sensitivity as defined here; but, for other supervisors it means knowledge of neurotic patterns and personal problems. If the supervisor assumes that the supervisee has deficits or problems that need remediation, then one approach to enhancing self-awareness will be taken. A different approach may be taken if the supervisor assumes that the supervisee has only areas that need strengthening. Personal awareness as a goal of supervision is different from personal awareness in psychotherapy in purpose, but in process they are often very similar. This distinction between personal awareness in supervision and therapy for supervisees is examined in detail in Chapter 4.

The functions of supervision and particularly the educative function form a basis on which specific goals can be achieved. The goals of professionalization, knowledge and skill acquisition, case conceptualization, and self-awareness are valued by professionals in all fields. The next step is to examine the process or means by which these goals can be attained.

SUMMARY

A global viewpoint has been taken throughout this chapter in order to highlight and clarify some of the terminology used throughout the fields of psychology, psychiatry, and social work. Of particular importance are the distinctions between the terms training, consultation, and supervision. These three processes are different in terms of the amount and type of participation by the persons involved and particularly by the sources of power used by the supervisor to promote learning.

Although the primary functions of supervision, in general, are supportive, administrative, and educative, further distinctions are made. The supportive function is viewed here as a necessary component of all forms of supervision. Administrative supervision focuses primarily on the administrative function and less on the educative function; clinical supervision centers mainly on the educative function and little on the administrative function. The educative function has been conceptualized as including the dimensions of knowledge of professional roles, clinical knowledge and skills, case conceptualization, and personal awareness. The focus of this text is on clinical supervision and how supervisors in training programs and in community agencies can become more effective in this task.

Chapter 2

A Conceptual Look at Clinical Supervision

THE SUPERVISORY PROCESS

Most supervisors probably have received a questionnaire from a student or a professional organization asking for the supervisor's model or theoretical framework for conducting supervision. Most supervisors, even experienced ones, would be challenged by such a questionnaire. Few supervisors have received formal training and even fewer have been given a conceptual framework for organizing their supervisory activities. Most supervisors begin their supervisory tasks by relying on memories of their previous supervisors and on their clinical approach to therapy as guidelines. One can imitate an outstanding supervisor, but without theory or a conceptual model one does not really understand the process of supervision.

Many supervisors have been forced to supervise without theoretical understanding and then form theoretical principles to follow. In essence every supervisor has been a theorist. As Hansen, Stevic, and Warner (1972) stated, "the theorist attempts to make sense out of life through the construction of a framework or model that allows him to explain events in a logical and reasonable manner" (p. 4).

One of the specific purposes of this chapter is to describe the dimensions on which supervisory behavior can be examined. These dimensions (functional relationship, hierarchy, and focus) have each appeared throughout the literature and are used in this chapter to help supervisors examine their own supervisory activities. A second purpose is to describe three models of supervision. Each model has a specific goal and within each model there is a wide choice of techniques to attain the goal of the model. The model used is based on three determinants. These determinants are supervisor characteristics, supervisee characteristics, and context characteristics. It is assumed that both beginning and experienced supervisors act on some framework. With some knowledge of models and the supervisory process, supervisors will be able to carry out their tasks with more consistency of purpose and with the confidence that comes from understanding.

Terminology

A model of supervision is the framework, which includes both the goal to be accomplished in terms of supervisee behavior, and the general behavior of the supervisor in attempting to accomplish the goal. The goal or desired outcome of each model of supervision is stated in terms of the ideal behaviors of the supervisee as a professional clinician. Each model contains a different description of important supervisee behavior to be attained. The statement of the supervisor's behavior consists of the functional relationship among participants, the hierarchy among participants, and the focus of the supervisor. These dimensions are examined in detail in the next section. *Techniques* are the specific supervisory interventions designed to encourage the supervisee to more closely approximate the ideal professional behaviors described within each model. Each model may be accomplished through many techniques. Some techniques may be used to carry out any model, whereas other techniques are idiosyncratic to a particular model.

Components of a Supervisory Experience

The face-to-face encounter between a supervisor and supervisee is a significant part of any total supervisory experience but should be considered in light of the other components of this experience (Hart, 1979). These components can be conceptualized as the what, when, and how of the experience, and are depicted in Figure 1. The "what" is content—what happens between supervisor and supervisee, such as in the supervisory model? The "when" is temporal application of the content—when does the supervision take place in relation to the supervisee's work with clients? Supervision may occur during the supervisee's session with the client (live), immediately following it (immediate), or at some later time (delayed). The "how" refers to the modality in which supervision is provided (i.e., individual, group, or peer sessions). Figure 1 illustrates, for example, how a supervisor could use group supervision immediately after supervisees had conducted counseling sessions (say, at the end of the day) and could employ either of the three models.

Content is described more specifically in Chapters 3, 4, and 5 and temporal application and modality are examined in Chapters 6 and 7.

Early Conceptualizations of the Supervisory Process

Until very recently, models of supervision have been ignored. Some authors described only goals and others described only processes, but few put these two concepts together to form models. The process of supervision has been typically described as didactic or experiential. The terms *didactic* and *experiential* have been used to describe supervision more frequently in psychology than other fields and were initially considered dichotomous. That is, supervision was viewed as either a didactic or an experiential process. Later, the idea of two separate but related variables (didactic and

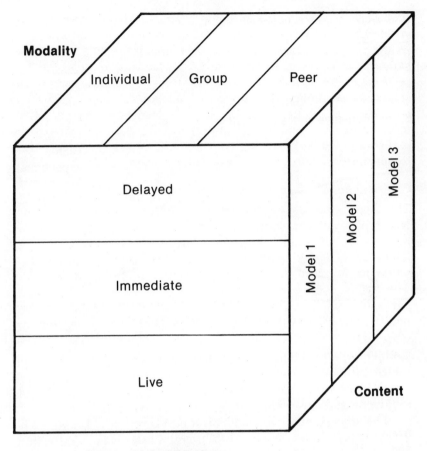

Temporal Application

Figure 1.   Components of a supervisory experience examined according to content, temporal application, and modality.

experiential) was generally accepted. In this latter conceptualization, supervision could be highly didactic, highly experiential, or somewhere in between. Figure 2 presents a visual comparison of these conceptualizations.

The terms *experiential* and *didactic,* in a strict sense, refer only to the behavior of the supervisor with no goal statement about the desired outcome of supervision in terms of the behavior of the supervisee. Consequently, these terms should be considered as general descriptors of supervision, not entire models. As used in this volume, the behavior of the supervisor using any model could be categorized as didactic or experiential depending on the partic-

A. A dichotomous conceptualization

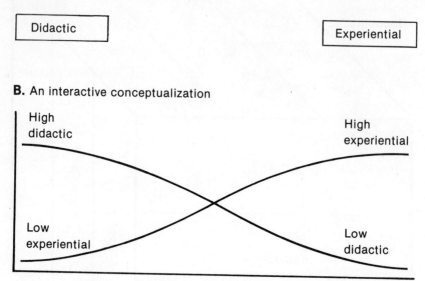

B. An interactive conceptualization

Figure 2.   Didactic and experiential conceptualizations of the process of supervision.

ular techniques used to accomplish the goal of the particular model. Figure 3 illustrates this position. Only three options per model are shown in Figure 3 but, as shown in Figure 2, many other blends of didactic and experiential techniques are possible.

The experiential "model" of supervision was described by D'Zmura (1964), Kaplowitz (1967), and Ekstein and Wallerstein (1972) and was clarified by Arbuckle (1963, 1965), Patterson (1964),

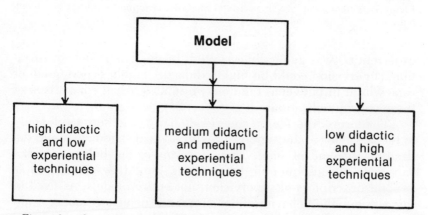

Figure 3.   Alternative supervisory techniques within a model of supervision.

Lister (1966a, 1966b), and Altucher (1967). They believe that the supervisor should focus on the supervisee's attitudes and feelings. The purpose of this supervisory behavior is to help supervisees understand and become sensitive to their own feelings as these feelings are displayed throughout interpersonal relationships. Supervisee awareness and understanding of these attitudes and emotions is regarded as a necessary condition for one to convey more effectively the therapeutic conditions of empathic understanding, unconditional positive regard, and genuineness.

The early experiential "model" is based on the assumption that supervisees need more insight and affective sensitivity than they already possess. Consequently, self-awareness of attitudes and emotions is thought of as a goal of supervision—different from other goals. This assumption is different from the assumption so often held in psychiatry that supervisees have neurotic patterns and personal problems that must be eliminated through supervision or personal therapy. Of course, psychologists, social workers, and others would agree that any supervisee with serious emotional problems should receive help but that a problem-oriented focus in supervision is inappropriate. Viewing personal awareness as an attribute to be developed or enhanced is the basis of the experiential "model" of supervision.

The didactic "model" was described by Mathews and Wineman (1953), Tarachow (1963), Dewald (1969), Semrad and Van Buskirk (1969), Windholz (1970), Spiegel and Grunebaum (1977) from the field of psychiatry and further defined by Krumboltz (1967), Delaney (1972, 1978), Butler and Hansen (1973), and Boyd (1978) from the field of psychology. In this model, the supervisor helps supervisees acquire specific techniques of counseling or knowledge of client behavior. The focus of the supervision session is the behavior (skills, interventions, techniques, or strategies) of the supervisee with a client and/or on the supervisee's understanding of a client's behavior.

The assumption of the early didactic "model" is that supervisees are in need of specific professional skills. Supervisees who demonstrate these specific skills thus indicate their professional competence. Competent therapeutic behavior, for example, is determined by an assessment of the supervisee's selection, implementation, and evaluation of appropriate techniques.

Both "models" are clear about their goals but narrow concerning the flexibility of the supervisor in accomplishing the goals. Supervisors who believed that skills were needed by the supervisee were subtly influenced to adopt a behavioral orientation to therapy. Conversely, supervisors who viewed supervisee insight and affective sensitivity as necessary, although not sufficient in many cases, felt as though they should be a phenomenological clinician. These ideas unnecessarily constrict supervisors and encourage competitiveness, which impedes development of supervision as a field of study.

A real breakthrough occurred when Truax, Carkhuff, and Douds (1964) and Carkhuff (1969) objectified therapist responses sufficiently so that these responses could be taught and measured. These responses were the ones that would convey the elusive therapeutic conditions necessary for client change. Affective responses by counselors now were taught in a didactic fashion. Other approaches have been developed, such as microcounseling by Ivey (1978), that apply a didactic teaching approach to phenomenological approaches to therapy. These and other approaches are described in more detail by Hart (1979).

Psychiatrists Fleming and Benedek (1966) also attempted a compromise between the didactic and experiential "models." They believed that the supervisor should use instructive approaches to increase a supervisee's skills and different approaches to increase supervisee's sensitivity to his or her attitudes and feelings. The application of either "model" is determined by the goals most appropriate to the developmental level of the supervisee. Overall, their compromise is one of using either "model" depending upon the needs of the supervisee. This position is significant because these authors believe that both skills and personal awareness of the supervisee are important and should be part of an ongoing and complete supervisory experience. Stated in this way, supervisors should consider the most appropriate goal for a supervisee at a particular point in the supervisee's development. Much can be learned from the examination of supervision in a longitudinal fashion.

A problem with Fleming and Benedek's position is that supervisors may infer that they must change their theoretical orientation to behavior change and therapy if and when they change goals with a supervisee. A clinician's therapeutic orientation is deeply rooted in personal beliefs and existing behavior patterns and would be difficult, if not impossible, to change significantly. Supervisors are advised to use the supervisory approach and techniques that are in agreement with their theoretical orientation to therapy but should be able to apply them to whatever goal is most important for the supervisee.

In conclusion, the early experiential and didactic "models" were helpful in initially showing differences in supervisory approaches.

Now concepts that are more inclusive need to be generated because supervisors do use a variety of affective and cognitive responses (Hamachek, 1971; Kadushin, 1974) in a variety of ways. Research by McElhose (1973), Smith (1975), Wilbur (1975), Newton (1976), and Wilbur and Wilbur (1979) indicate the complexity and range of supervisory behavior that exists. Clustering supervisory behavior into a single didactic-experiential continuum does not show the complexity of the behavior. As Nash concluded from her factor-analytic study of supervisory behavior, "The therapeutic [experiential]-didactic polarity, despite its importance in the literature, is not a useful way to conceptualize actual supervisory situations" (Nash, 1975, p. 40).

To obtain a precise description of the process of supervision, supervisor behavior could be measured by the number of statements used by the supervisor that are designed to produce cognitive or affective responses in supervisees. How often and under what conditions particular supervisory statements should be used are unanswered questions. Research that moves supervision into a position that considers goal attainment and approaches in a more independent fashion will be particularly helpful in understanding the process of clinical supervision.

DIMENSIONS OF SUPERVISION

The dimensions of supervision described in this section were derived by a deductive approach. From an examination of many supervisors, supervisors-in-training, and supervisees, plus a thorough review of the research and descriptive literature in psychology, social work, and psychiatry, three dimensions have been isolated by which the process of clinical supervision can be differentiated. The dimensions that form the basis for the conceptual models of supervision presented in this volume are:

1. The functional relationship between supervisor and supervisee
2. The hierarchy between supervisor and supervisee
3. The focus of the supervisory session

Functional Relationship

The *functional* relationship between the supervisor and supervisee does not refer to the emotional quality of their relationship. The function of their relationship refers to how the supervisor and supervisee work to attain the goal of supervision as illustrated by what they communicate rather than how they feel about each other.

Each person makes statements during supervision illustrating how each of their behavior patterns fits or compliments the other's.

The concept of complementary interpersonal relations has been developed by Leary (1957) and applied to psychotherapy by Haley (1963). These authors believe that all interpersonal relations can be assessed by the complementary ways in which the participants act toward each other. In an analysis based on communications theory, Haley (1963) differentiates complementary relationships from symmetrical relationships. In a complementary relationship "the two people exchange behavior which complements or fits together. One is in a 'superior' position and the other in a 'secondary' position in that one offers criticism and the other accepts it, one offers advice, and the other follows it, and so on" (Haley, 1963, p. 11).

Balsam and Garber's (1970) description of the characteristics of supervisors most desired by supervisees further clarified the concept of functional relationships. In their factor-analytic study five factors emerged that described the primary characteristics of psychotherapy supervision as reported by psychiatric residents. Three of these factors defined the emphasis of the supervisor and were labeled 1) psychodynamic aspects of supervision, 2) clinical management, and 3) group therapy. Two factors defined the personal style of the supervisor as seen by supervisees and were termed 1) warm, and 2) active. Two fusion factors emerged that defined types of desired supervisors. The first factor combined warm and active, and was labeled "interested teacher" by the researchers because the supervisor was concerned about the supervisee and engaged in a didactic supervision process. The second fusion factor was composed of psychodynamic aspects of supervision and warm and was labeled "admired clinician." This supervisor was also interested in the supervisee and particularly in the development of the supervisee's "clinical sensitivity." The combination of certain supervisor behaviors, for example, expressing interest in supervising plus the value of supervisor behavior by supervisees, shows that specific functional relationships, for example, admired teacher and interested clinician, exist and are significantly different from each other.

Functional relationships have also been described in the writings of Nash (1975), Nelson (1978), and particularly by McElhose (1973). McElhose (1973) showed that supervisor-supervisee dyads could be distinguished according to what he termed *behavioral complementarity,* and suggested that this factor is an important component of effective supervision.

Three patterns of relationships emerge from the many descriptions of supervisor-supervisee relationships. One pattern is that of teacher and student; second is therapist and client; and third is collaborators. Each of these relationship patterns is determined by a particular goal of supervision. Each model of supervision has a different goal or goals; therefore, the function of the supervisor and supervisee will differ with each model.

Teacher-Student Relationship This supervisor believes that theory, techniques or professional positions must be conveyed to the supervisee. This goal puts the supervisory dyad into a teacher-student or an "apprentice-master" relationship (Schuster et al., 1972, p. 168). The supervisor takes the position of having some skill and knowledge to convey to the supervisee who does not have this information and must have this information to become a competent professional clinician.

Therapist-Client Relationship A supervisor may believe that a supervisee must gain self-awareness of attitudes and feelings, and so the supervisory relationship takes on a therapist-client stance as in a therapeutic relationship. Ekstein and Wallerstein (1972) stated that to gain increased psychotherapeutic skill a supervisee must develop in "the use of oneself in a therapeutic relationship" and that the development may be "far-reaching and deep" (p. 138). Supervisors who adopt the goal of personal awareness will use their clinical skills to help supervisees learn about themselves in terms of becoming aware of their general interpersonal behavior and their feelings in those interpersonal interactions. The assumption underlying this goal is that supervisees who have greater personal awareness will be better clinicians.

Collaborative Relationship One additional relationship pattern occurs when a supervisor believes that a supervisee has sufficient skills and/or personal awareness and now must integrate these two dimensions into more effective professional practice. This integration puts the dyad into a colleague relationship in which the supervisor serves as a collaborator with the supervisee with respect to the supervisee-client interaction.

Each of the three relationship patterns described here relies on a positive emotional relationship between supervisor and supervisee. Gale (1976) reported that the quality of teaching by psychiatric supervisors as perceived by supervisees is affected by the quality of their relationship with their supervisors. When the quality of teaching by psychiatric supervisors was rated *good* by supervisees, rapport was also rated good. Some of the supervisees who rated their rapport with their supervisors as *poor*, however, still rated the teaching as *good*. One can speculate how good the teaching might have seemed to this latter group had a better rapport existed.

The rapport or emotional relationship between supervisor and supervisee has been most frequently assessed in terms of facilitative conditions such as empathy, genuineness, and concreteness (Carkhuff, 1969). Experimental research in psychology shows that supervisors who demonstrate high levels of empathy, regard, genuineness, and concreteness toward supervisees produce supervisees who exhibit these same qualities (Pierce & Shauble, 1970, 1971a, 1971b). Perhaps the results are attributable to the modeling process; but whatever the cause, the emotional relationship of supervisor and supervisee does produce certain behavior by the supervisee.

The relationship between facilitative conditions offered by supervisors and the positive reactions/evaluations by supervisees has been largely accepted by many practioners. A highly facilitative supervisor will certainly be more effective than a supervisor low in facilitative conditions. Some of the early research, however, relied on the assumptions of the experiential "model" and implied that facilitative conditions by the supervisor are not only necessary but also sufficient to produce competent practitioners. Studies comparing methods of teaching supervisees to convey facilitative conditions to clients show clearly that only supervisory modeling of facilitative conditions is not as effective as structured and didactic methods (Payne & Gralinski, 1968; Payne, Winter, & Bell, 1972; Goldfarb, 1978). The level of facilitative conditions offered by supervisors is best conceptualized as a dimension on which all clinical supervision is based but one that is not sufficient for effective supervision.

Research on facilitative conditions in supervision implies that high levels of facilitative conditions preclude other expressions by the supervisor. Research by Blumberg and Amidon (1965), Blumberg (1968), and Oratio (1977), however, shows that supervisors who are high in facilitative conditions and are directive and critical are still rated high in effectiveness by supervisees. Supervisees of these facilitative and critical supervisors also attain high levels of therapeutic gains with clients. As supported by Lambert (1974) and Leddick and Bernard (1980), the emotional aspect of the supervisory relationship is an important but separate part of the overall supervisory relationship.

Finally, research on the effects of facilitative conditions conveyed by supervisors is frequently measured only in terms of facilitative conditions offered by supervisees to clients. Unfortunately, some supervisors reading this research believe that communication of facilitative conditions is a sufficient skill for counselors to have. This position oversimplifies the process of therapy. Hansen, Pound, and Petro (1976), in their review of research on supervision in psychology, concluded that "although teaching facilitative communication is necessary, it is not sufficient; research on supervisory procedures that improve other counselor skills is needed" (p. 114). The emotional and the functional relationship are both important components of the supervisory process. Further research may help to determine the effects of both of them on supervisees.

Hierarchy

Hierarchy in a supervisory relationship refers to the superior position that the supervisor has over the supervisee. Although some (Ackerman, 1973) believe that egalitarian relationships are possible, the majority favors the idea stated by Haley (1976) and others that hierarchy is always present between supervisor and supervisee. This superior position is based on the type and amount of power the supervisor uses in order to influence the supervisee. The type of power is determined initially by the characteristics of the supervisor such as organizational position and expertise as indicated by academic degrees, awards, or years of experience and later, as the supervisory relationship develops, on the identification of the supervisee with the supervisor.

A primary determinant of hierarchical distance is the supervisee's perception of the supervisor's characteristics and behaviors in the supervisory session. It is suggested here that supervisees who perceive the supervisor's characteristics and behavior as vastly more competent than those of the supervisee will have a greater *hierarchical distance* than supervisees who perceive less distance between the competence of themselves and that of their supervisor. A large hierarchical distance between supervisor and supervisee strengthens the role of the supervisor as teacher or master clinician and, correspondingly, the role of supervisee as student or novice. As the distance increases, the roles become more clearly differentiated, thereby strengthening the expectations of supervisor and supervisee to respond to each other in a complementary fashion (Haley, 1963).

Given the assumption that the hierarchy between supervisor and supervisee is not an absolute but is a quantity determined by perceptions of both persons, the hierarchical distance can and does differ between various supervisor and supervisee dyads. For example, a supervisor (Dr. Neal) and his or her supervisee (Mr. Carr) have perceptions of the hierarchy between them that differ from the perceptions of the hierarchy between Dr. Neal and her other supervisee (Mr. Elwin) even though both supervisees are similar in years of experience, level of training, skills, and personal awareness. In the first supervisory dyad Dr. Neal and Mr. Carr may perceive a great distance between themselves, and in the latter, Dr. Neal and Mr. Elwin may perceive much less distance between themselves. The reasons of either supervisee or supervisor for these perceptions may vary widely according to the personality of the particular individuals and the context in which the supervision is conducted.

Research support for differences in hierarchical distance is provided by McElhose (1973) who found that various supervisor-supervisee dyads differed in terms of what he called "relational distance" as determined by analyzing the content of supervisory sessions. Therefore, it is suggested that a supervisor in any model of supervision establishes a large hierarchical distance by conveying that the supervisee is less professionally or personally competent than the supervisor. This message is communicated by a supervisor's critical observations, expressions of doubts about a supervisee's basic abilities, excessive interpretations about the supervisee's or the client's behavior, unclear, mystical, or cryptic statements about psychotherapy, or lengthy disclosures about brilliant clinical successes of the supervisor. The supervisor's motivation may be to establish and maintain greater distance, to gain feelings of competence or superiority, to control the supervisee or (at worst) to punish the supervisee. More appropriately, the supervisor may wish to maximize his or her impact on the supervisee.

Supervisees also contribute to greater hierarchical distance by eliciting evaluative and directive comments from the supervisor, adopting a self-deprecating posture, telling only errors and disappointments, or asking the supervisor to share exciting success experiences. Some supervisees may seek to establish a large hierarchical distance in order to justify or validate their feelings of inferiority or incompetence. Others may seek protection from the results of possible clinical errors by elevating their supervisor to an unrealistically high level of competence or even to a position of omnipotence.

Supervisors and supervisees may attempt to reduce the hierarchy between each other. A supervisor may accomplish this by encouraging a supervisee to have confidence in his or her own ideas, skills, and sensitivity, to try out new approaches, and to convey that the supervisor's ideas are not necessarily superior to those of the supervisee. A supervisee may establish a low hierarchical distance by operating more independently and relying less on the supervisor for directives. A supervisor's motivation to achieve this low distance might range from a desire for emotional closeness and colleagueship to fear of his or her own power and authority. A supervisee might want this reduced hierarchical distance for reasons such as fear of authority figures and a rejection of them to a desire to become a more independently functioning clinician.

Hierarchy is the structural arrangement of people—one above the other—usually according to variables commonly accepted as salient to professional work such as skill, experience, years of training, and position or role within the organization. Other variables not so readily accepted as salient, such as race, sex, or physical appearance, are also likely to contribute to hierarchical distance. Variables such as these remain relatively constant. Once a hierarchical distance is established, the only variable subject to change is the perceptions of those variables, and perceptions change as the result of the behavior of both supervisor and supervisee. McElhose (1973) found that hierarchical distance changed during the middle 10 weeks of a 30-week supervision experience. An example of a supervisor's increasing hierarchical distance is when Ms. Talmidge, a supervisee, begins supervision with Dr. Franklin, who she has heard is an excellent diagnostician, therapist, and theoretician. During the first few supervision sessions, Ms. Talmidge made a request for feedback about some specific skills and Dr. Franklin agreed to this arrangement. Dr. Franklin then critiqued her every word in a clinical session he had viewed on tape, offering many alternative approaches and techniques that could have been used and describing how successful these techniques have been for him. Also, Dr. Franklin predicted the behavior of Ms. Talmidge's client for the coming week as a result of Ms. Talmidge's work. Dr. Franklin elevated himself to a higher level by his wealth of suggestions and predictions.

It is further believed that hierarchical distance is related to the model of supervision a supervisor implements. Supervisors and supervisees using a particular model of supervision engage in behaviors that are appropriate for that model and that establish a certain hierarchical distance. When using a different model, the same supervisor and supervisee will behave somewhat differently because the goal of the model is different, thus establishing a greater or lesser hierarchical distance. Using the research format of McElhose (1973), supervisors may be able to decide if an optimum hierarchical distance exists and how this distance can be established.

Focus

Focus of the supervision session refers to the person or persons toward whom the supervisor directs the discussion. Grotjahn (1955) described *patient-focused* (dynamics of the client and skills of the supervisee) and *supervisee-focused* (general attitudes and feelings of the supervisee) supervision. Fleming (1953), Fleming and Benedek (1966), and Gaoni and Neumann (1974) also wrote about these two types of focus of supervision, and Rosenbaum (1953) added *process-focused*. Process-focused refers to the discussion of the patient's transference toward the therapist, that is, the patient-therapist relationship.

In a factor-analytic study of psychiatric residents and psychology trainees by Nash (1975), supervisors focused on one of three main areas. One area was a personal, career focus. In this focus the supervisors were open, and they encouraged openness by the supervisees. They also socialized the supervisees into the profession by sharing experiences and defining terms used within the profession. Although the relationship between supervisor and supervisee is discussed, the supervisor does not focus on the supervisee's knowledge, techniques, or relationship with specific clients. A second area is a therapy-relationship focus in which the supervisors helped supervisees examine relationships with specific clients, especially their feelings toward clients. The third focus was on conceptualizing the dynamics of specific clients with no exploration of the supervisee's feelings toward the client or techniques to implement.

In this volume, focus is directed toward the content of what the supervisor and supervisee discuss. There seems to be some justification for thinking of one main focus on the technical and conceptual skills of supervisees in their interactions with specific clients, a second more personal exploration of the general concerns of supervisees about themselves and their development, and a third focus on the relationship between supervisees and clients.

THREE MODELS OF SUPERVISION

By combining the dominant goals and processes described in the literature on supervision, three models of supervision can be formulated. In addition, these formulations are based on the work by

Hart (1974, 1978) and Hart, Maslin, Liberi, and Wondolowski (1976a, 1976b, 1976c). Videotapes illustrating these models were produced by Hart (1976a, 1976b, 1976c). Similar formulations of models of supervision, developed by Kurpius and Baker (1977) and Boyd (1978), are mentioned here for clarification of terms.

The goals of the *Skill Development model* of supervision are to increase the technical skills of the supervisee with clients and to increase the supervisee's conceptual understanding of clients. This model is referred to as a teaching model by Kurpius and Baker (1977), but the term *teaching* is imprecise because it could refer to everything that supervisors do using any model of supervision. The functional relationship between supervisor and supervisee, however, is certainly that of a teacher and student in that the supervisor has knowledge and skills that the supervisee does not possess. The supervisor then conveys this information to the supervisee. The hierarchical distance between supervisor and supervisee is relatively large because of the expert power (French & Raven, 1960) used to influence the supervisee in the learning process. The focus of the session is usually on the client's problems, background, behavior patterns, and motivations followed by a focus on the supervisee's techniques to help the client.

The *Personal Growth model* is similar to the therapeutic model described by Kurpius and Baker (1977), and Boyd (1978). "Therapeutic," however, connotes therapy, thus creating confusion as to whether a therapeutic model of supervision is really therapy and not supervision at all. "Personal growth" implies an emphasis on the development of the supervisee as a person without the probing, uncovering, and remediation that occurs during therapy. A complete discussion of the differences between the Personal Growth model of supervision and psychotherapy is presented in Chapter 4.

The goal of the Personal Growth model of supervision is to increase the insight and affective sensitivity of the supervisee. Insight is defined as knowledge of one's interpersonal behavior patterns. Affective sensitivity refers to awareness of emotions that occur within the supervisee during interpersonal interactions. The functional relationship of the supervisor and supervisee in the Personal Growth model is that of counselor and client. The supervisor is more insightful and sensitive than the supervisee, and has the skills to help the supervisee gain more insight and affective sensitivity. The hierarchical distance is usually moderate but can range widely depending on the behavior of the participants. The power used by the supervisor is typically a combination of expert power and referent power depending on the amount of the supervisee's identification with the supervisor. The focus of the sessions is on the supervisee's personal feelings and thoughts about interpersonal relations, which are generally aroused by his or her interaction with a client, and has, unlike therapy, an educative not a problem-resolution emphasis.

The goal of the Integration model is to help supervisees integrate their acquired skills and personal awareness into effective relationships with clients. The ideal clinician in this model is one who can relate to clients with spontaneity and consistency and has a clear idea of motives and intentions for behavior in professional relationships. These goals are usually to be attained after the supervisee has gained basic skills and knowledge by means of other models of supervision. Researchers such as Kurpius and Baker (1977), Gurk and Wicas (1979), and Littrell, Lee-Borden, and Lorenz (1979) have used the term *consultative* to describe this model. Consultative supervision is a reasonable term except that it is too easily confused with consultation, a process that is different from supervision as shown in Chapter 1.

The functional relationship between supervisor and supervisee is that of colleagues (Mosher & Purpel, 1972, p. 144) or collaborators. Both persons are viewed as having knowledge and expertise that are applied to the analysis of the supervisee and client interaction and to the supervisor-supervisee interaction. The hierarchical distance between supervisor and supervisee is small because the supervisor does not emphasize the differences in expertise or organizational position.

The primary focus in the session is on the supervisee-client unit, which is seen as an interactive dyad. This view differs from the typical linear view of a supervisee input and client response. The supervisee-client relationship in the Integration model is seen as circular because both persons affect the actions of the other. A secondary focus is on the supervisor-supervisee interaction as it affects and is affected by the supervisee-client interaction. The effects of these two interactions upon each other is referred to as parallel process.

The Skill Development, Personal Growth, and Integration models of supervision, when compared in terms of the three dimensions—the functional relationship between supervisor and supervisee, the amount of hierarchical distance between supervisor and supervisee, and the focus of the supervision sessions—yields the matrix shown in Table 1.

Table 1. A comparison of the skill development, personal growth, and integration models of supervision according to functional relationship, hierarchical distance, and focus

	Skill Development model	Personal Growth model	Integration model
Functional relationship	Teacher-student	Counselor-client	Collaborative
Hierarchical distance	High	Moderate	Low
Focus	Supervisee's skills with and understanding of the case	Supervisee's self-insight and affective sensitivity	Supervisee's integration of skills and personal awareness as demonstrated in the supervisee-client interaction

The amount of hierarchical distance according to model is best expressed as both a range and a typical distance within that range. In the Skill Development model the distance between supervisor and supervisee ranges from high to moderate. The typical hierarchical distance in this model is probably higher than the typical distance in either the Personal Growth or Integration models. The range of hierarchical distance in the Personal Growth model is high-to-low depending on the particular supervisor-supervisee combination and typical distance is probably between the Skill Development and Integration models. Finally, the range of hierarchical distance in the Integration model is moderate-to-low, with a typical distance being low. Typical hierarchical distance in the Integration model is lower than in either the Skill Development or Personal Growth models.

DETERMINANTS OF THE MODEL USED

Supervisors should deliberately choose a model of supervision on an examination of three interdependent variables: 1) the characteristics of the supervisor, 2) the characteristics of the supervisee, and 3) the characteristics of the context in which supervision is conducted. Schuster et al. (1972), in a comprehensive review of supervision in psychiatry, believes that these "basic elements of the supervisory situation must be brought in explicit focus" (p. 72). Supervisors will become more effective if they clearly and purposefully use a model of supervision selected according to these three elements; supervision should not be a random process.

It is believed that most supervisors do not consider their own characteristics, the supervisee's characteristics, or the context characteristics before beginning supervision except in the most visceral way. Supervision is not examined by supervisors because most of them have had no formal, informal, or inservice training in supervision. Consequently, the characteristics of the supervisor, supervisee, and context have an unpredictable impact on the model that is implemented and may lead to a supervisor switching models with little forethought. By examining these characteristics, supervisors can begin to understand the variables that influence their choice of a model of supervision and with this understanding may make choices that lead to more positive effects on supervisees.

A final reason for considering the characteristics affecting the model used is so that the field of supervision can be better understood. With this understanding, more adequate theories can be constructed. In this way, supervision can become a process to be learned—a science more than an art.

Supervisor Characteristics

The characteristics of the supervisor refer to those aspects of the supervisor's personal and professional background that influence the choice of a model of supervision. The characteristics chosen for examination and deemed most salient are the supervisor's 1) training and experience, 2) interpersonal style, and 3) theory of psychotherapy.

Supervisor's Training and Experience   The supervisor's clinical training program and how supervision was viewed during this training affects the supervisor's choice of a model. Training programs that emphasize skill acquisition may encourage clinicians, who later become supervisors, to adopt this same view. Also, goals of training programs may differ among the fields in the mental health area. For example, psychiatrists may choose a particular model more frequently than will social workers or psychologists because of the differences in goals of the training programs each group experienced. Survey research comparing professional groups and the dominant model they use, if any, would be extremely valuable.

A specific aspect of training would be the particular type of supervision one received. As has been frequently stated in the social science literature, a clinician's application of therapy skills is influenced by one's supervisor. For example, 13 psychiatric residents at San Francisco's Langley Porter Neuropsychiatric Institute reported that "Although we felt that the process of arriving at a theoretical orientation and mode of therapy was determined primarily by our personalities, we sensed that the kind and type of resident-supervisor relationship played an important role" (Fleckles, 1972, p. 150). In an analogous way, a new supervisor's model of supervision may be influenced by the model used by his or her supervisor during training or work. For example, a clinician who received supervision via a Personal Growth approach and found supervision valuable might use the same model as a supervisor. Of course, this supervisory experience is affected by the number and quality of supervisory experiences a clinician received, both during training and on the job. A testable hypothesis, however, is that the more positively a clinician identifies with a particular type of supervisory experience (model used and/or supervisor as a person) the more the clinician will duplicate that experience later as a supervisor.

In addition to training, the extent of a supervisor's experience as a supervisor is also important. An experienced supervisor will be able to assess the effects of the selected model of supervision on a variety of supervisees who work with a variety of clients. The more experience in terms of numbers and types of supervisees, the more information a supervisor will have on which to evaluate the model of supervision chosen.

Supervisor's Interpersonal Style   The supervisor's own stylistic relationship patterns affect the choice of a model in that some supervisors learn more and feel more comfortable in, for example, a didactic relationship. Other supervisors learn more and gain more satisfaction when engaging students or workers in a more colleague-like, or personal, relationship. The specific interpersonal characteristics such as extroversion, need for structure, insecurity, anxiety level, or dogmatism that may influence one's choice of a model have not been determined. Furthermore, few supervisors are likely to have examined their interpersonal patterns and then made a conscious choice of a model. The selection process is probably quite intuitive. One of the most important contributions to understanding the supervisor's motivations in using particular approaches and techniques was contributed by Schuster et al. (1972). In addition to their excellent review of supervision literature of psychiatry, these three supervisors recorded their seminar discussion with psychiatric residents on the topic of supervision. Their thoughts provide an inconclusive yet rich and intimate portrayal of the strong influence of the supervisor's style of relationship patterns on the choice of a model of supervision.

Supervisor's Theory of Psychotherapy   Another influence on the supervisor's selection of a model of supervision is the supervisor's theory of psychotherapy. Liddle and Halpin (1978) and Liddle (1979) believe, as does Patterson (1964), that one's basic assumptions about behavior change are the same when applied to either supervision or therapy. This assumption seems quite valid and would lead to the belief that supervisors who adhere strictly to a particular therapeutic orientation such as a behavioral, cognitive, or psychodynamic theory would use the model of supervision that most agrees with the assumptions of their theory of therapy more often than models whose assumptions do not agree with those of their therapeutic orientation. The suggestion has been made that a supervisor who has a behavioral or cognitive approach to therapy would adopt the Skill Development model and that a psychodynamic clinician would adopt the Personal Growth model. This position is tenable except for two issues.

One issue that makes the direct relationship between one's clinical orientation and one's model of supervision less clear is the fact that many supervisors are eclectic in orientation thereby using, for example, a psychodynamic theory in the early stages of therapy and a behavioral theory later on in the process. Most clinicians are probably eclectic and so would be likely to use two or more models of supervision depending on the supervisee and the context in which supervision is being conducted.

An additional issue is that clinicians of various theoretical orientations to therapy find all the goals of skill development, personal growth, and integration to be important for supervisees but that some goals are more important than others and therefore deserve more emphasis. This belief leads clinicians with a behavioral or cognitive orientation, for example, to supervise only supervisees not needing or wanting personal growth, which is unlikely to occur, or to focus primarily on skill development and secondarily on personal growth and integration, which is what probably happens in actual practice. It is believed here that a supervisor's orientation toward therapy interacts with one's choice of a particular model of supervision but does not determine the model of supervision in a strictly linear relationship. A supervisor who is a phenomenologist, for example, will conceptualize in phenomenological terms, but this supervisor may use these conceptualizations to improve supervisee's techniques with clients, to increase the insight and affective sensitivity of the supervisee, or to achieve some integration between techniques and personal behavior patterns. The decision about what goal to accomplish (and thus what model to use) is dependent upon consideration of the supervisee's needs and the context in which the supervision is offered. For example, Ms. Lottes, a supervisor with a Rogerian orientation, says to Bob, her supervisee: "Well, Bob, I think you might be even more supportive of Karen's attempts at independence. You've never quite explored how good she feels when she's on her own. And also you might bring up with her how good she seemed to feel last month when she made the decision to take the night school course." Apparently, Mrs. Lottes believes in a phenomenological approach to counseling, as her choice of words suggests, but she is quite instructive about her supervision, which suggests the use of the Skill Development model.

In the next example, Mr. Rankin, a supervisor with a behavioral orientation, says to his supervisee, Ellen: "Ellen, I'd like to see you give more verbal reinforcement to Karen during your counseling sessions—particulary about her efforts at going out in the evenings and calling friends to make social arrangements. Since Karen sees you as a powerful person in her life, you'll be able to do shaping that may extend outside your sessions." Mr. Rankin uses behavioral terms to describe the counseling process, and he is didactic in his approach, which is characteristic of the Skill Development model of supervision.

Both Ms. Lottes and Mr. Rankin apparently view the supervisee as needing assistance in using an approach with a particular client and so the Skill Development model is appropriate. The fact that Ms. Lottes, a Rogerian clinician, does not make comments that are high in warmth, empathy, and genuineness merely means that she has assessed the supervisee as needing specific skills instruction.

Conversely, if a supervisor with a behavioral orientation to therapy decided that a supervisee needing some understanding of frustration or disappointment over failure with a client, the supervisor might use a series of questions designed to pinpoint the specific reasons and cause for these feelings. Then, the supervisor might use cognitive restructuring to reduce the unpleasant feelings and their debilitating effects, if any, and then plan for the future in which similar situations might occur. In this instance, the supervisor consistently uses a behavioral approach toward behavior change but the goal is clearly within the Personal Growth model.

To gain a more complete understanding of the relationship between therapeutic orientation and model of supervision, research should be conducted on groups of clinicians/supervisors who maintain particular therapeutic orientations to determine whether a relationship exists. Survey or field research of a correlational nature as suggested here has many disadvantages, but in an area such as supervision, many exploratory questions must be answered before more definitive experimental investigation can be conducted (Goldman, 1976; Gelso, 1979).

Supervisee Characteristics

The supervisee influences the choice of a model of supervision by coming to supervision with an expectation about what goal should be accomplished and how this goal should be attained in terms of supervisor behavior. Supervisee expectations are based on the supervisee's 1) prior training and experience as well as 2) learning pattern.

Supervisee's Training and Experience   The training program of the supervisee may influence expectations of what is needed in order to be a competent professional. Clinicians from social work may have different expectations of their supervisors than psychologists have of their supervisors. These expectations would be communicated, directly or indirectly, at the outset of supervision thereby causing a reaction by the supervisor.

The supervisee's past experience with supervision is also important insofar as expectations toward the present supervisor are concerned. Articles with the supervisee's point of view by Miller and Oetting (1966), Barnat (1973), Gaoni and Neumann (1974), and Gale (1976) suggest that a supervisee's evaluation of prior supervisory experiences strongly shapes subsequent supervisory relationships.

Supervisee's Learning Style   Perhaps the most important aspect of the supervisee in terms of the choice of model is the supervisee's learning pattern. Learning pattern is viewed by some in terms of supervisees' characteristics such as level of cognitive complexity (Berg & Stone, 1980) or in terms of teaching approach of the supervisor such as deductive or inductive. At this point a great deal of survey research is needed to determine the supervisee characteristics that most affect their learning and the teaching approaches that have the greatest long-term impact on supervisee performance.

At another level supervisee learning patterns may be viewed in terms of the supervisee's reaction to a skill development versus a personal development emphasis in supervision. It seems that some supervisees have a clear preference for one emphasis or the other in terms of what helps them at a particular point in their development. Supervisors who help supervisees to determine the most helpful emphasis and then provide that emphasis may be individualizing the learning process in a very effective way.

Context Characteristics

The third determinant of the model of supervision, and perhaps the most difficult to assess, is the characteristics of the context in which the supervision is provided. Context refers to the setting where supervisors and supervisees conduct their clinical work. For practicing clinicians, the setting would be their place of employment, and for students, the setting would be their field work or internship site. Every setting influences both supervisor and supervisee. Sources of these influences include: 1) operational procedures of the organization, 2) expectations of administrators, and 3) the client population served by the organization. The listing of these sources of influence does not suggest a simple linear relationship between these sources and the supervisory process but rather a complex interrelated whole in which each part influences all other parts. Perhaps the complexity of this relationship has deterred all but a few authors in the mental health field from examining context.

Williamson (1961) discussed the importance of context on social work supervision; yet, Schuster et al.'s (1972) thorough review of psychiatric literature produced only Emch's (1955) article on context and supervision. The influence of researchers in organizational development and systems theory as applied to psychotherapy and of social scientists such as Bateson (1979), however, have led to closer examinations of context on supervision and training.

Operational Procedures   One source of influence on staff members, frequently described in the organizational development literature (Cartwright & Zander, 1953; Collins & Guetzkaw, 1964), is the operational procedures of the agency. Certain procedures cause emotional reactions—disappointment, frustration, anger— among students or staff members who are restricted in some way. As more clinicians experience this distress, staff morale declines and effective service to clients also diminishes. A supervisor may be the first person to witness the emotional reactions of the supervisee and so has an opportunity to work with the supervisee on the specific procedure over which the supervisee is upset.

Administrators' Expectations   The expectations by administrators of the staff have an impact on supervision. These expectations are important in that agency administrators may desire certain ends to be accomplished through supervisory activities. For instance, they may wish to have staff develop skills or strengthen overall staff morale. Awareness of administrative wishes could encourage supervisors to choose a particular model that would best carry out the goal of the administrator. For example, when an administrator and supervisor agree that certain skills are generally weak among the staff, the supervisor might adopt a Skill Development model of supervision to increase the needed skill. Conversely, an agency director who observed low staff morale might suggest that supervisors use a Personal Growth model to help students or staff resolve feelings of disappointment or frustration.

Another aspect of the context is the tasks clinicians perform. Kadushin (1976), citing Wasserman (1970) and Arndt (1973), stated that in social work agencies "Stress can result from the nature of social work tasks and the conditions under which the work is done" (p. 217). In some agencies, mental health professionals are assigned very specific tasks such as assessment or treatment planning or career counseling. In other work settings a person is expected to be a generalist who can perform a wide variety of tasks. Whether the supervisee is expected to be a specialist or a generalist will affect the choice of a model of supervision. Furthermore, a specialist who may have already attained a high level of skills can now focus on personal growth; consequently, the Personal Growth model is needed. Or a competent generalist may now wish to focus on specific skills needed for a particular assignment, which would suggest the use of the Skill Development model.

Client Population   One additional characteristic of the context as an influence on supervision is the client population served by the agency. For example, a supervisee who works with clients who are psychotic, severely physically handicapped, extremely poverty-stricken, or substance abusers is likely to face frustrations and fears to a degree that a supervisee with different clients may not experience. Such students or staff, understandably, could be expected to have a higher-than-average need for supervision centered on feelings. A very careful examination of the services offered by the agency and the clientele served by the agency is needed in order to understand this aspect of the context variable.

The effects of context on the actual practice of clinicians has been examined to a limited extent. For example, Sharaf and Levinson (1957) and Kurtz and Kaplan (1968) showed that psychiatric residents are influenced in their choice of treatment approaches by the ideology of the training center. Similarly, residents are affected in their use of chemotherapy by ward staff (Chin-Piao & Appleton, 1970) and by their peer group including ward staff and residents (O'Connor, 1965). The effects of context on the model of supervision used, however, is just now being examined. The description of the influences within a particular setting gives an overview of the subtle yet powerful impact of the context in which supervision is conducted.

The combination of context with supervisor characteristics and supervisee characteristics results in the likelihood that a certain model of supervision will seem to be more appropriate than others. By being sensitive to these three variables, supervisors can choose the model of supervision with the greatest potential for success.

SUMMARY

Supervision has advanced from the early conceptualization of didactic versus experiential to the point where more explicit models can now be constructed with some degree of confidence. Based on the research in psychology, psychiatry, and social work, three distinct models are proposed here—each with a different goal for the supervisee to attain. These models are called Skill Development, Personal Growth, and Integration.

The characteristics that most clearly differentiate these models are the functional relationship between supervisor and supervisee (teacher-student, therapist-client, or colleagues), the hierarchical distance between them, and the focus of the session (supervisee knowledge of and skills toward the client, personal awareness of the supervisee, or the relationship between supervisee and client). These characteristics are the components that when combined in particular ways produce a model that can accomplish particular goals for supervisees.

Furthermore, these models may be applied by means such as individual, group, or peer sessions or at various times (with respect to the supervisee's clinical sessions with clients) such as delayed, immediate, or live. Of primary importance in the choice of a model and the manner in which it is applied are the characteristics of the supervisor, such as training; of the supervisee, such as learning style; and of the context, such as administrators' expectations. With careful consideration of these characteristics, a supervisor can choose a model of supervision that will bring about maximum learning for each supervisee.

SECTION II

MODELS
OF CLINICAL
SUPERVISION

Chapter 3

Skill Development Model

DESCRIPTION OF THE MODEL

GOALS
  Case Conceptualization
  Skill Acquisition

CASE STUDY

TECHNIQUES
  Case Notes
  Psychological Report
  Role-playing
  Sitting-in
  Observation
  Audiotape and Videotape Recording
  Coaching
  Co-therapy
  Group Work
  Peers

APPLICATION OF THE SKILL DEVELOPMENT MODEL
  Guidelines
  Evaluation

SUMMARY

DESCRIPTION OF THE MODEL

Although the Skill Development model is based on the earlier didactic "model," it has been expanded, making it truly a model and not just a description of a teaching approach or supervisory techniques. Kurpius and Baker (1977) describe models this way: "Models have goal orientations and seldom prescribe or imply any technique for achieving a goal" (p. 227). Therefore, the Skill Development model is named for an overall goal rather than a process, such as didactic or teaching, to accomplish that goal.

The Skill Development model has two distinct goals that are to help supervisees conceptualize diverse aspects of cases and to acquire specific therapeutic skills to be used with these cases. These goals are thought by some supervisors to be the only goals appropriate for supervision (Haley, 1974), although other supervisors believe these goals to be necessary but not sufficient (Barton & Alexander, 1977).

Most supervisors adopt the Skill Development model for a large part, if not all, of the supervisory experience for either students or practicing clinicians. Perhaps the most compelling reason for using this model is that desired performance of the supervisee can be clearly specified and assessed. Viewing supervisee performance as skills to be learned, although threatening, makes it possible for the process to be accomplished, given the appropriate learning conditions.

The approaches to accomplishing the goals of the Skill Development model can vary. Kadushin (1976) remarked, "Most supervisors apparently use a mix of expository direct teaching and dialectical-hypothetical indirect teaching procedures. Expository teaching amounts to 'telling'; dialectical-hypothetical teaching involves questions and comments which help the supervisee find his own answers" (p. 168). Indeed, the Skill Development model encompasess a variety of teaching approaches by supervisors with a variety of orientations to therapy.

A supervisor's teaching method and orientation to therapy influence the approach used to accomplish the goals of the Skill Development model. Consequently, a supervisor could use the techniques listed in this chapter and still maintain a particular orientation to teaching and therapy. Of course, there will be some consistency between a supervisor's approaches to teaching and therapy, as Liddle and Halpin (1978) suggest.

Of the three models of supervision presented in this volume, the Skill Development model is the easiest to understand and apply because its characteristics are so objectively defined and described. The model is differentiated here in terms of the three dimensions described in Chapter 2: 1) the functional relationship between the supervisor and supervisee, 2) the amount of hierarchical distance between the supervisor and supervisee, and 3) the focus of the session.

The functional relationship established between supervisor and supervisee in the Skill Development model is that of teacher and student. The supervisor accepts a superior role to the supervisee in terms of clinical expertise. Conversely, the supervisee accepts the role of learner. The relationship allows the supervisor to question the work of the supervisee and to make requests of the supervisee. The supervisee, in turn, asks for the supervisor's analyses and evaluations of the supervisee's work and suggestions for techniques to be implemented. Both supervisor and supervisee agree that the supervisee can learn most efficiently and effectively by the supervisor's imparting of knowledge about client behavior and effective clinical practices.

The second factor differentiating models of supervision is the extent of the hierarchical distance between supervisor and supervisee. In all models of supervision the supervisor is, to some degree, in a higher position than the supervisee, resulting in a greater or lesser hierarchical distance between them. In the Skill Development model, typically there is more distance between the supervisor and supervisee than in the other models of supervision. The distance in the Skill Development model, however, can vary from a low amount (as in guide to traveler) to a high amount (as in Guru to disciple) (Ferber, 1972). Some supervisors and supervisees seek a relatively low amount of distance between them and others seek a high amount of distance. Some supervisees who want low hierarchical distance seek a supervisor whose techniques and interpersonal behavior deemphasize the hierarchy between them, and other supervisees who want a high amount of distance select a supervisor whose techniques and behavior increase the hierarchy. It is important to note that a supervisor may use words that seem to establish a low amount of hierarchical distance such as, "I *suggest* that you . . ." or "*Consider* using a technique such as . . ." or "*Perhaps* what you *might* do is . . ."; however, upon examination of a longer supervisor-supervisee interaction, this supervisor clearly establishes a high degree of hierarchical distance through evaluative terms and specific suggestions or interpersonal behavior described in Chapter 2. Research must include consideration of the supervisor's intent with respect to hierarchy and the impact on supervisee learning.

The focus of the Skill Development model is on the supervisee's understanding of the client and the effective application of that understanding through appropriate techniques. The specific ideas and skills discussed depend on the perceptions of the supervisee and the supervisor of the client with whom the supervisee is working. The supervisor assumes that the supervisee has some knowledge and skills already acquired through more formal means or through experience. The appropriate application of knowledge and skills, however, requires a highly individualized learning process. The Skill Development model is implemented when the supervisor, as part of an overall training program, with input from the supervisee, decides that information and skills are needed to assist the supervisee in working with clients.

The Skill Development model can be used when the supervisor and supervisee discuss either a specific client or a type of client the supervisee faces. For example, the supervision session might center on a client whose behavior in the clinical sessions or out of the sessions is difficult for the supervisee to understand. One supervisee, Ms. Tucker, had difficulty understanding the lack of motivation of a young black mother of two children who was divorced and on welfare. Ms. Tucker, who was also black and divorced but middle class, lacked understanding of the client's passive, aimless, and emotionally-detached behavior. A discussion of the effects of poverty and inadequate education was undertaken in supervision within the Skill Development model that helped Ms. Tucker better understand her client. Similarly, the supervisor of Mr. Warner responded to statements of concern by Mr. Warner about several clients who had displayed similar patterns of aggressive behavior with their spouses. The supervisor used the Skill Development model to help Mr. Warner more clearly understand the meaning of aggressive behavior among couples and then to examine various techniques to help such clients. In each example, an individual client or several clients with similar patterns, the supervisor used the Skill Development model appropriately and effectively.

In the Skill Development model the supervisor and supervisee function as teacher and student; hierarchical distance between them varies but tends to be considerable; and their supervisory sessions focus on the supervisee's work with particular clients. The goals toward which supervisors more specifically direct their attention are addressed in the next section.

GOALS

The two goals of the Skill Development model are 1) to help the supervisee conceptualize aspects of present cases and 2) to acquire specific therapeutic skills to be used with clients. These two goals correspond to the conceptual and executive skills described by Cleghorn and Levin (1973) in addition to perceptual (observational) skills. Although the case conceptualization and skill acquisition goals are divided here for purposes of clarification, both are valued equally and should be acquired during the course of supervision. A supervisor using the Skill Development model typically will work on both goals within each session because both are mutually dependent on each other for maximum clinical effectiveness of the supervisee.

Case Conceptualization

The goal of case conceptualization is based on the assumption that a clinician will be more effective with a clear case conceptualization than with one that is unclear. Although authors like Carkhuff (1969) have supported skill training with little emphasis on case conceptualization, most supervisors believe that a greater degree of understanding of the client's behavior and its causes aid the clinician in working with the client. Consequently, most supervisors using the Skill Development model begin with case conceptualization and later move to skill acquisition.

Case conceptualization as a goal in the Skill Development model is characterized by discussions between supervisor and supervisee aimed at increasing the supervisee's understanding of the behavior of a client or type of client. Discussions encompass the client's general and specific behaviors, motivations, needs, underlying personality dynamics, interpersonal style, reinforcers, or any other useful means of describing and comprehending the client.

The supervisor also helps the supervisee understand client behavior in terms of labels and descriptions previously learned in the classroom. Even though supervisees have learned the definitions of various behaviors and labels, they may not be able to identify the behavior of clients as presented in clinical sessions. By discussing the behaviors of the client displayed in a therapy session or reported by the client as occurring outside the session, the supervisee can form a personal lexicon of terms to describe behavior. Labels such as neurotic, depressed, or self-defeating may be selected from a variety of theoretical orientations. Any theoretical orientation is acceptable in the case conceptualization approach as long as the orientation is thoroughly understood and mutually agreed upon by both supervisor and supervisee. When the supervisee's orientation to therapy differs from that of the supervisor, new supervisory dyads may be needed if maximum supervisee learning is to take place. Other possible solutions are discussed in Chapter 7.

A central part of achieving the case conceptualization goal is the gathering of isolated facts about the client's behavior and forming these facts into a framework that is useful to the supervisee in selecting approaches and techniques for helping the client to change. The supervisor and supervisee discuss, for example, the social and medical history of the client, results of psychodiagnostic testing, records of schools or other agencies with whom the client has been involved, and anecdotal reports written by other mental health workers who have previously seen the client. This discussion helps the supervisee establish a complete profile of the client. It is believed by supervisors using this model that effective clinical techniques are decided after thorough examination of available information about the client.

A specific part in attaining the case conceptualization goal is a discussion of what maintains the negative, self-defeating, or unwanted behavior of the client. Here the supervisee must move from what is objectively known about the client's behavior to the cause for the continuation of the client's behavior. The supervisor and supervisee must use their knowledge of theory and their collected facts to describe the possible internal and external causes of the client's behavior. From this description the supervisor and supervisee decide on appropriate procedures for helping the client. Then a supervisor and supervisee can discuss general strategies that could be used with a client such as individual counseling, group, or family counseling. Other strategies could include diagnostic testing, consultation with other agencies, use of medication, hospitalization, or referral.

Skill Acquisition

The skill acquisition goal of the Skill Development model of supervision refers to the discussion between the supervisor and supervisee of the general treatment strategies and specific therapeutic techniques to be implemented by the supervisee with a particular client or type of clients. The skill acquisition goal is often characterized by suggestions from the supervisor of treatment strategies, critiques of the supervisee's techniques, demonstration of techniques by the supervisor, and practice of techniques by the supervisee (Worthington & Roehlke, 1979). Although all of these supervisory activities are not used by all supervisors, they are mentioned here to illustrate the variety of activities that effectively meet this goal of supervision.

Another activitiy is to discuss the theoretical approaches to therapy such as client-centered, Gestalt, or behavioral preferred by the supervisee. The supervisor helps the supervisee in the application and evaluation of this approach. Several potential difficulties can arise at this point. One difficulty can occur when a supervisee has a theoretical orientation that is unfamilar to the supervisor; yet the supervisor tries to be helpful in a general way. The supervisee may receive less than adequate supervision in the Skill Development model because the supervisor, who is supposed to be an expert, is not an expert in this theoretical orientation to therapy. To compound the difficulty, some supervisors will not discuss cases or techniques within the framework of the supervisee, thus forcing the supervisee to adopt a new framework or else give lip-service to the supervisor's orientation. These difficulties are discussed in more detail in Chapter 7.

In addition to discussing general strategies that supervisees may use with clients, supervisors focus on specific techniques or interventions that superviseees may use with clients. Examples of such clinical techniques include confrontation, reflection of feelings, systematic desensitization, interpretation, dream analysis, empty chair, and behavior rehearsal. The supervisor may suggest a particular intervention, demonstrate it, give instructions on its use, have the supervisee practice it, as well as give instruction on criteria for selection and evaluation of a particular type of technique. The selection, application, and evaluation of general strategies and specific therapeutic techniques are all part of the process designed to achieve the skill acquisition goal of the Skill Development model.

Both case conceptualization and skill acquisition are important in supervision, especially for beginning students or workers, because they may have read about a type of client or a technique or have seen them demonstrated on film but have not actually encountered such a client or tried the technique. After developing a clear case conceptualization based on available data, supervisor and supervisee decide on appropriate therapeutic strategies such as individual, group, or family therapy and therapeutic goals within a particular theoretical orientation to therapy. Then, as therapy proceeds, the supervisor critiques and corrects the supervisee's specific therapeutic techniques. The case study given below illustrates how one supervisor worked to attain the case conceptualization and skill acquisition goals of the Skill Development model.

CASE STUDY

The following case study illustrates typical responses of a supervisor using the Skill Development model of supervision. The case is taken verbatim from *Styles of Supervision III*, a videotape developed by Hart (1976c) and the *Instructor Manual* for the videotape written by Hart, Maslin, Liberi, and Wondolowski (1976c). The comments in the left-hand margin note the points at which the supervisor illustrates one of the following dimensions: 1) the functional relationship of the supervisor and supervisee, 2) the hierarchical distance between supervisor and supervisee, and 3) the focus of the session.

Comments	Supervisor-Supervisee Interaction

	Supervisor:
	    Beth! Hello. Sit down.
	Supervisee:
	    Hello. Thank you.
	Supervisor:
	    Well, how have things been going?
	Supervisee:
	    Just fine, just fine.
	Supervisor:
	    Good. Did you have a particular case you wanted to talk about this week?
	Supervisee:
	    Yes. I want to talk with you some more about Joe, because I'm a little bit frustrated on exactly what direction to head with him.

Supervisor focuses on the client	Supervisor:
	    Sure. Joe, now, you'll have to refresh me. Joe was . . .
	Supervisee:
	    Joe was the one who is just really afraid of failing. His grades are not improving in spite of working with him all this semester so far. And because he failed before he is afraid of failing a second time, which would have a sort of double stigma to it. And he may fail—he's right on the borderline.
	Supervisor:
	    He really *isn't* performing.
	Supervisee:
	    Right. He's not performing, and the last time that . . .

Comments	Supervisor-Supervisee Interaction
	Supervisor: He was, what, seventh grade, was it? Supervisee: Right. And the last time I viewed him in a classroom situation he was still having a lot of problems getting down to work, and snapping out of daydreaming or thinking about whatever he was thinking about, and really cooperating with the classroom activity; he was just very slow and tired looking . . .
Supervisor checks on the extent of data gathering on the client by the supervisee	Supervisor: Right. Now, as I remember, you had already canvassed the teachers, and you'd gotten teachers' comments, and that kind of thing. I can't remember, had you interviewed the family? Did you get some background and developmental history on him? Supervisee: I spoke with the father on one occasion, but that was on a very . . . just kind of an accident meeting, and I didn't get that kind of information from him then. His mother came into school, his stepmother came into school on a separate occasion a couple of weeks later, and I spoke with her, but not to a great extent; she was concerned also about his grades and she had come to the school to speak with his teachers specifically, which she did, she spoke to them . . . Supervisor: I see, yeah. So you haven't had a real chance to investigate to see if there might be some information in the background that might be helpful to you. Supervisee: Exactly. I could have asked his stepmother except that she's recently married his father, so she really doesn't know Joe very well at all. Supervisor: She doesn't know Joe, uh huh. Supervisee: But she is concerned about his school grades and would like to do something about that.

Comments	Supervisor-Supervisee Interaction
Supervisor checks another source of data that the supervisee should use	**Supervisor:** Yeah. Did the elementary school teachers, if you look in the records, you know, did they have any comments that were helpful? **Supervisee:** Uh, the teacher comments that I saw, looking at his background in elementary school and up to this date, are pretty much the same, that with a lot of help and a lot of extra work, he can come up to par, but he needs continual encouragement, it's like he needs somebody behind him to prod him, he just isn't. . . .
Supervisor points out consistency of reported data	**Supervisor:** Um hum, so they've been saying the same thing, pretty much? **Supervisee:** Exactly. He just can't do it on his own. He seems to have difficulty.
Supervisor probes for supervisee's knowledge of causes for client's behavior in order to facilitate a clear conceptualization of the case	**Supervisor:** Yes. And they don't give you any clues as to what underlies this? And they tell you what the behavior is but you still have no. . . . **Supervisee:** I'm waiting . . . nothing there.
Supervisor reduces hierarchical distance by asking for supervisee's opinion about an approach	**Supervisor:** Uh huh. Now is this something you *want* to find out—do you think it would be important to know what the underlying causes might be? **Supervisee:** Yes. I've been trying to work with him about that, as you know, discussing why he's being depressed, what he thinks about when he daydreams in class, and trying to get that and discuss that a little bit more. But, uh, ...
Supervisor evaluates the supervisee's approach in terms of the effect on the client	**Supervisor:** How have the results been? **Supervisee:** Well, I've gotten a lot of information, but he's still having trouble in class. He

Comments	Supervisor-Supervisee Interaction
	has improved a bit with some teachers, but it's kind of a day-to-day battle, and there is not a marked improvement.
	Supervisor:
	Right. It's still a puzzle to you.
	Supervisee:
	Right, right.
Supervisor suggests another source of data on the client	Supervisor:
	Do you think that some kind of psychological evaluation might uncover some information that would solve this puzzle for you?
	Supervisee:
	Um hum. I hadn't thought about that, but that might be a good idea.
	Supervisor:
	Yeah. If there's a waiting list and all that, but if you think that it's needed, why go ahead and put in your request. Now, in the meantime, has there been any other agency involvement with this family during the time when they had no mother present and all that—do you know if there might be any information available from the social agency?
	Supervisee:
	Not that I know of. He used to live with his grandmother before his father remarried, so that he was being taken care of within the family, but I don't know of any agency intervention at all.
Supervisor shifts to treatment planning and clearly shows the functional relationship—teacher and student	Supervisor:
	Well, it's worth checking, and maybe the nurse's office would be another ... check the medical record and so forth. Gather up all the information that you can—it might lend, it might shed some light on this, to get to the root of it. In the meantime, have you set up some goals that you feel perhaps are reasonable, that you might accomplish with him before the end of the year?
Now the supervisor looks at skill development, specifically the supervisee's goals.	
	Supervisee:
	I think the most immediate goals, the most pressing ones, are for him to try and improve his grades, and in order to improve his grades, he's going to have to improve on a day-to-day level, as far as class participation, and doing what is

Comments	Supervisor-Supervisee Interaction
	expected of him as far as homework and in-classroom work. And if we could just start improving that, maybe the grades could. . . .
Supervisor's focus is on supervisee's techniques and encourages low hierarchy via a question instead of a command	**Supervisor:** So there are really two areas where you need to change his behavior—one is in the classroom, and one is work at home. Right. Now, have you been thinking about how you might approach this? You want to effect behavior change. . . .
	Supervisee: Right. Well, so far I've been working with his teachers in a behavior modification sort of scheme. And that has helped to a certain extent, but I don't want him to become dependent on getting rewards every day and looking for that sort of thing . . .
	Supervisor: Oh, you're afraid of that, I see.
	Supervisee: . . . so that when that falls off, he, you know, he won't cooperate with the teachers any more.
	Supervisor: Yes.
	Supervisee: I don't know, I have this feeling.
	Supervisor: You're afraid that external incentives will rob him of internal incentives?
	Supervisee: Exactly, exactly. So I'm trying to phase out of that without having him drop off completely and relapsing into a total daydreaming sort of scheme of things.
Supervisor acts as a teacher by suggesting a change in the technique to be used	**Supervisor:** Perhaps you can think of some kind of reinforcement that won't be so obvious, so that they will have the effect but he won't be dependent on them because he may be less conscious. Do you think that's possible?
	Supervisee: Do you have some suggestions?
	Supervisor: Well, what I'd like you to do is come up with a program that we could concentrate on if you will detail one

Comments	Supervisor-Supervisee Interaction
	day's behavior in a classroom, and maybe we can work on that as a model and see how we can maybe restructure the behavior mod. program so that you won't have that concern. We'll try that, anyway. Do you think it's worth working with the family in any way, Beth?
	Supervisee:
	I think it would be. First of all, he's fortunate because he has two parents who are interested in his progress at school and would like to help him in some way.
Supervisor is the source of evaluation for the supervisee	Supervisor:
	Good, I'm glad that you found that out. That's a good thing to establish.
	Supervisee:
	Yes. Both of them have come to school on separate occasions, on his behalf. And that indicates to me that they are very interested, and they have said as much to me. I'm just unsure.
	Supervisor:
	Now how can you use this—here you've got a resource, how can you use that?
	Supervisee:
	Exactly. How can I use them as....
	Supervisor:
	Yes. All right, now, one thing you're concerned about is his homework. That is pulling his grades down, evidently. Is that it?
	Supervisee:
	I think he made some attempts, he just doesn't get it all done.
	Supervisor:
	Okay, can you also set up a behavior mod. program with his parents?
Supervisee responds as a student or novice Supervisor gives guidelines about implementation of an approach (Supervisor as expert and supervisee as novice)	Supervisee:
	How would I go about doing that?
	Supervisor:
	Okay, well, you know essentially how to do it, but the things to watch out specially for, I think, are to make sure the parents know what the goal is, for the desired behavior. If their behavior, if their expectations are out of line, you *know* that it won't work, right? So, you'll have to be very clear about that. I

Comments	Supervisor-Supervisee Interaction
	think if you get this data together, and we sit down next week, and maybe we can put together a program for home and a program for classroom.
	Supervisee:
	Okay.
	Supervisor:
	Now were there any other cases that you wanted to talk about today?
	Supervisee:
	Yes, there was one other one that I wanted to bring up, there's been some problems that have developed within the past week.

The supervisor in the preceding case study used only a few of the many available techniques. In the next section techniques are described that are most commonly used within the Skill Development model of supervision.

TECHNIQUES

Case Notes

In many social work agencies and other mental health facilities, reviewing case notes is the main supervisory technique. Typically, case notes consist of the supervisee's impressions of what occurred in a particular session with a client. Specific kinds of information and the form to be followed vary with the supervisor's preference and the agency procedures. One form for reporting on a session with a client may be found in *Practicum Manual for Counseling and Psychotherapy* (Dimick & Krause, 1975) or in the description by Hewer (1974). After the supervisee has written out the data in the appropriate format, this information is reviewed in the supervision session. The supervisor uses this information as a basis for focusing on case conceptualization or skill acquisition.

Case notes, like the psychological report described next, help the supervisee concentrate on the behavior of the client and the clinical interventions used in a particular session. Because the notes are written after the clinical session and before the supervision session, the supervisee has sufficient time for thought and reflection on what happened in the clinical session. This time can be used profitably by the supervisee in conceptualizing the case and evaluating treatment strategies and techniques used with the client.

A practical advantage of the case notes technique is that several clients can be reviewed within a single supervision session, which allows the supervisor to maintain a degree of control over client welfare and allows the supervisee to feel more protected from making an unrealized error. Case notes can serve as valuable indicators of progress with clients—a welcome aid to busy supervisors.

A drawback of this technique is that case notes are not an exact description of what happened in the clinical session, and are only a partial and sometimes distorted representation. The most conscientious supervisee will find it impossible to recall and relate all the significant verbal and nonverbal elements of the interaction during a therapy session. Those supervisors who wish to accurately perceive what the client does and how the supervisee and client interact will be dissatisfied with a review of case notes. They must use more objective forms of data reporting such as audiotape or videotape review, or direct observation.

Psychological Report

A very effective technique in case conceptualization is the assimilation of data from many sources to form an informal or working psychological report. The "report" is a verbal picture of the client based on information gained from sources in addition to the supervisee's initial interview with the client. These sources include psychodiagnostic testing, work samples, medical reports, educational background, anecdotal reports from family and friends, and observations from mental health professions in other agencies. The supervision session would be devoted to helping the supervisee learn where to look for information, how to obtain it, how to assimilate it, and how to develop a treatment plan for the client based on the report that is formed.

In many cases a wealth of information is available, but supervisees do not know where to find it. Sometimes information may be needed that is not available except through consultation with another professional, as in the case of a psychodiagnostic or physical examination. Supervisors can assist supervisees in knowing when additional information should be gained and where to obtain the information. In addition supervisors must assist supervisees in learning the appropriate procedures for obtaining information about a client. For example, the supervisor must discuss with the supervisee the professional manner in which confidential information should be requested.

Once the information is obtained, the job of assimilating it can begin. This task is often overwhelming for supervisees because of the large quantity of collected information. The heart of the case conceptualization approach, however, is a thorough analysis and synthesis of information about a client. As each bit of information is examined, two major questions must be asked: 1) How does this particular fact relate to the other facts already known? 2) How do the facts already gathered help to decide on an approach to take with the client (a treatment plan)? The supervisor's expertise as a clinician is used extensively with the supervisee in answering these questions.

The use of a working psychological report to aid supervisees is important by itself and in combination with other supervisory techniques. Following the establishment of a comprehensive report including approaches for the supervisee to implement with the client, the supervisor can now help the supervisee to learn the specific skills associated with carrying out an approach.

Role-playing

Role-playing is the least complex and most effective supervisory technique in the Skill Development model to help supervisees acquire specific skills. The purpose of role-playing is to provide supervisees with understanding and confidence in using a particular clinical technique. The primary assumption of role-playing is that specific skills can be acquired quickly and precisely through actual observation and practice, not just through discussion. Furthermore, for a supervisee who may have failed in an attempt to use a technique with a client, role-playing can aid in future implementation of that technique. Another assumption is that the supervisee will be less anxious with the supervisor than with the client and in this low-threat atmosphere, will learn a technique more effectively than through trial-and-error learning with a client. An additional rationale for using role-playing or any skill-acquisition technique is that of ethical responsibility. Professional codes of ethics discourage the use of clinical techniques with clients without prior training through supervised simulation activities such as role-playing.

Two ways of role-playing used most frequently are: 1) supervisor-as-clinician, supervisee-as-client, and 2) supervisee-as-clinician, supervisor-as-client.

When the supervisor is the clinican and the supervisee is the client, two goals are present. The first goal is for the supervisor to understand the client's concerns and typical behavior. By taking the role of the client the supervisee demonstrates these concerns and behaviors. After a portrayal of a few minutes, both supervisor and supervisee react to the client (as portrayed by the supervisee) and comment on the relationship between the supervisee's verbal descriptions of the client and the supervisee's portrayal of the supervisee.

Because the emphasis is on the supervisee's view of the client in a global sense, the specific content of what the supervisee (client) says is largely irrelevant. The supervisee can portray any of the client's concerns and display any of the client's typical emotional responses. Also irrelevant, at least initially, are the supervisor's (clinician's) interventions during the role-play. Discussion following the role-play would center on the supervisee's view of the client in order to increase both the supervisee's and supervisor's understanding of the client.

The second goal of the supervisor-as-clinician, supervisee-as-client role-play is to teach the supervisee to use a particular clinical strategy. The supervisee adopts a particular client mannerism or problem, then observes how the supervisor-as-clinician responds. This procedure is based on the premise that the supervisor is an expert clinician and can share this expertise with the supervisee by overt demonstrations. Following the role-play, the supervisor and supervisee discuss the technique used by the supervisor so that the supervisee clearly understands the purpose and desired outcome of the technique.

The supervisee then duplicates the technique. The supervisor plays the client and the supervisee portrays the clinician and uses the technique demonstrated earlier by the supervisor. In the discussion following this supervisor-as-client, supervisee-as-clinician role-play, the actions and skills of the supervisee are critiqued by both the supervisor and the supervisee. Following this critique, another role-play could be conducted for additional practice by the supervisee.

A valuable adjunct to role-playing is recording the interaction on audiotape or videotape. The supervisor and supervisee can review the tape together in the supervision session to aid in conceptualization or skill acquisition. Furthermore, the tape is available for the supervisee to review following the supervision session in order to reinforce the learning that took place.

Role-playing is applicable to a wide variety of techniques and is an effective tool for supervisors. Of course, the effectiveness rests on the accuracy of the supervisee's understanding of the client, the skill of the supervisor, and the ability of both supervisor and supervisee to simulate the clinical setting. Naturally, role-playing is artificial but practicing a technique with some sense of realism will help a supervisee to be able to duplicate the technique in actual therapy sessions.

Sitting-in

A technique mentioned more frequently in the literature of psychiatry than that of social work or psychology is sitting-in (Schuster & Freeman, 1970). In this technique, the supervisor sits in the room with the supervisee and a client as the supervisee conducts a clinical session with the client. The purpose of this technique is to provide the supervisee with support and an occasional corrective comment if needed. Discussion between the supervisor and supervisee typically follows the clinical session with the client.

In this technique, the supervisor becomes a relatively inactive observer who intervenes to give advice to the supervisee or to address the client directly. Some supervisors prefer to let the supervisee make all of the interventions, offering some suggestions to the supervisee but no comments to the client. In this way the supervisee clearly has primary responsibility for the client. Conversely, some supervisors act as a junior partner to the supervisee, making interventions directly to the client in order to direct the supervisee or to illustrate what the supervisor believes to be an innovative or highly effective strategy. A supervisor might vary the degree of direct intervention while sitting-in, depending on the supervisee's preference and the client's responsiveness.

Sitting-in is most often used at the beginning of clinical work with a particular client and usually lasts for only one session; it is typically limited to the initial interview segment of a supervisee's work with a client such as an intake interview, a testing session, or history-taking session.

As supervisees become more skilled and knowledgeable, supervisors use sitting-in less frequently. Furthermore, the increased use of one-way observation mirrors and tape recordings makes sitting-in less necessary. Sitting-in is probably used best with those beginning students who have high anxiety about working with clients and need the support of a supervisor to make the transition from classroom to clients. An alternative technique is for the student to sit-in but not participate in clinical sessions conducted by an expert clinican to observe the interventions with a client. In this way, a novice can become more confident and learn certain approaches and skills to be used in the future with other clients.

For more experienced supervisees, the supervisor may sit-in with the supervisee for a single session. This consists of a consultation of sorts, which allows the supervisee to get unstuck or to have the supervisor better understand the client and the supervisee's approach. The use of the supervisor for sitting-in allows for a temporary but powerful use of a supervisor's clinical expertise. Afterward, the supervisor and supervisee discuss the clinical session.

A discussion of the performance of the supervisee and/or conceptualization of the client or both is usually held after the sitting-in session. This discussion is especially important for beginning supervisees to ensure that they clearly understand the intent of the suggestions made by the supervisor to the supervisee during the clinical session and the interventions made directly by the supervisor to the client.

Observation

Observation of a supervisee by the supervisor from behind a one-way mirror is significantly different from the case notes or sitting-in techniques. In the case notes technique, the supervisee has a considerable degree of independence from the supervisor because the supervisor has no first-hand knowledge of the clinical session. Furthermore, the supervisee has maximum control of the session because the supervisor does not actually view the supervisee's behavior. In the sitting-in technique, the supervisee has less independence and control than in the case notes technique because the supervisor now has direct knowledge of the clinical session and opportunity to direct the session. Observation permits the supervisor to view the clinical session directly yet allows the supervisee independence and control of the session. For many supervisors and supervisees the observation technique is an effective compromise between the case notes technique and the sitting-in technique.

Observation is used best when adequate preparation occurs before the clinical session takes place. Prior to the session, the supervisor and supervisee should review the background of the client and the approach and techniques used previously with the client. Specific goals for the session should be discussed. The supervisee should inform the supervisor of any items the supervisee wants the supervisor to observe and evaluate. This pre-observation session is most clearly delineated by Goldhammer (1969), Cogan (1972), and Reavis (1978) as an important step in the process of clinical supervision. With thorough preparation, the observation session can be effective in enhancing supervisee knowledge and skill.

During the observation of a clinical session, most supervisors take some form of notes. A detailed scale for rating a clinician's behavior was developed by Hackney and Nye (1973). Note-taking is advisable because of the large amount of information produced during the session. Some supervisors record verbatim comments made by the supervisee or the client for use as illustration during the post-observation conference with the supervisee. Other supervisors record global impressions of the behavior of the supervisee, the client, or the interaction between them. The form of the notes can vary as long as they are directed to the points discussed in the pre-observation conference.

Following the observation, a supervision session should occur where the supervisor reacts to the observed behavior of the supervisee. Usually, this session occurs immediately following an observed clinical session. In this session the supervisor points out errors and strong points, discusses the supervisee's conceptualization of the client as a result of the clinical session, and considers what new approach or techniques, if any, should be used in the future. It is helpful for supervisees to keep the supervisor's notes made on the clinical session for later review.

A helpful modification of the observation technique is to have multiple observers as described by Hare and Frankena (1972), Tucker, Hart, and Liddle (1976), Papp (1977), and Tucker and Liddle (1978). Multiple observers can be used in one of two basic formats. During the clinical session, the observers can verbalize their observations to the supervisor who then uses this information in the post-observation discussion. In this format, the observers can be completely honest in their observations because they do not have to face the supervisee directly. The supervisor chooses the information to be conveyed during the feedback session with the supervisee and structures the amount and type of feedback into words that can be heard and can be helpful to the supervisee. In the second format the observers and the supervisor all meet with the supervisee for a post-observation session. Although the supervisor can deliver all of the feedback, the observers typically offer their own observations with the supervisor providing some direction (Tucker et al., 1976). This format certainly involves the observers to a greater extent than in the first format, which is an advantage if the supervisor is a skilled group leader and can use this "group" format to advantage.

Audiotape and Videotape Recording

Increasingly, supervisors find audiotape and videotape recordings of supervisee performance with clients to be the most useful technique of those used in the Skill Development model of supervision.

Over the last 30 years, audiotaping has been available to clinicians as a means of recording an exact account of what took place. No longer does a supervisor need to wonder about the difference between the supervisee's memory of a session and what actually happened in that session. With the advent of videotape, nonverbal as well as verbal communication can be assessed, and a more complete analysis can be conducted of the supervisee's conceptualizations and skills (Schiff & Reivich, 1964). Clinicians in some professions, however, have been slow to use audiotape and videotape. Kadushin (1976) commented, "the use of such procedures is becoming widespread in human service professions generally, despite its current limited use in social work" (p. 419). Perhaps the use of audiotape and videotape recordings is slow in becoming popular because of the lack of generally accepted procedures for using the tape recordings.

Empirical research in counseling and clinical psychology consistently shows effective results in using audiotape and videotape for feedback to students. Walz and Johnston (1963) reported that counselors changed their perceptions of themselves and their clients after viewing a videotape of their counseling sessions. Additional work by Kagan, Krathwohl, and Miller (1963), Markey et al. (1970), and Kagan (1975) support the idea that clinicians can gain knowledge and skills by reviewing audiotapes or videotapes. Only a few authors, for example, Berger (1970), Rhim (1976), and Meltzer (1977), however, describe guidelines needed by supervisors to use tape recordings effectively.

Choosing Audiotapes or Videotapes   Assuming that both audiotape and videotape equipment is available, one of the primary decisions is which type of recording to use. Research in psychology by Beiser (1966), Markey et al. (1970) and Ward, Kagan, and Krathwohl (1972) has failed to show significant differences in effectiveness of audiotape compared to videotape feedback as measured by supervisee performance of skills. Perhaps differences between these two means of feedback are attributable to the phase of supervisee development or to differences in certain emotional or intellectual characteristics of the supervisees.

Although differential effects of audiotape and videotape for feedback purposes is unclear, research on the preferences of supervisees provides some logical direction. Descriptive research shows that supervisees prefer to receive audiotape feedback at the beginning of their training program and videotape feedback later on (Yenawine & Arbuckle, 1971), but the specific reasons for these preferences are not given. Poling (1968a, 1968b) suggested that greater anxiety occurs among supervisees when given videotape feedback compared to audiotape feedback. Part of the reason for greater anxiety is probably due to embarrassment over viewing oneself. Anxiety is also likely because of the overwhelming amount of data a supervisee receives when viewing a videotape (Stoller, 1968). Supervisees can spend an entire supervision session on one or two segments of a videotape because of the tremendous amount of information the tape recording has provided. A logical suggestion for using tapes is, therefore, to use audiotapes in early supervision sessions and introduce videotapes after initial anxiety of the supervisees has diminished. In this way supervisees will become adept and comfortable with audiotapes before using videotapes. An additional method of preventing undue supervisee anxiety is for the supervisor to be well-trained in the use of audiotape and videotape feedback. Consequently, the supervisor can react to supervisee anxiety without an overemphasis that stems more from the supervisor's fears about supervisory competence than the supervisee's fears about clinical competence.

A variation from the procedure of using audiotapes first and videotapes later is to have the supervisee listen to an audiotape of a clinical session and then view a videotape of the same session (Poling, 1968b). With this method the supervisee has fewer cues on the audiotape and so is less likely to be overwhelmed compared to viewing a videotape. After reviewing the audiotape and the videotape prior to the supervision session, the supervisee is more comfortable in working with the videotape in the supervision session. Once a sequence is established, specific clients can be designated for taping.

Selecting Clients to be Taped   Two options exist in deciding who should be taped. In the first option the supervisee tapes a variety of clients so the supervisor and supervisee can review the range of the supervisee's skills. The assumption made by the supervisor is that supervisees must learn to select techniques and modify them according to the unique characteristics of clients. Clients selected for taping often are chosen because of their differences such as personality, problems, age, race, and sex in order to provide the supervisee with a wide range of experience. In order to accomplish this differential application of techniques, a supervisee will tape many clients. This allows the supervisor to check on the supervisee's flexibility and judgment in the application of skills. As the supervisee progresses, new and perhaps more difficult clients will be assigned to the supervisee for taping. A further reason to have supervisees tape most, if not all, of their clients is to monitor the overall quality of service given to the clients.

In the second option, the supervisee tapes only one or two clients with whom clinical work had just begun and continues to tape these clients until their termination. By using the same client throughout the course of supervision, both supervisor and supervisee can focus on supervisee knowledge and skills without adjustments for different clients. The supervisee will be able to understand the beginning, middle, and termination of the clinical process by following a single client through the three phases of the process. Research and thoughtful consideration are needed in order to help supervisors make an appropriate choice of either the multiple client or single client approach.

Preparing for Supervision   Typically, a supervisee will make an audiotape or videotape of a session with a client and bring the tape to the supervision session for review. The tape is played with the supervisor or supervisee stopping the tape to comment on a particular interaction between supervisee and client. The supervision session will cover as much of the tape as can be played and discussed in the time allotted. Many modifications of this standard procedure exist that improve the efficiency and effectiveness of supervision with tape recordings.

One important procedure for improving the effectiveness of using tape recordings is that the supervisee listens to the tape before the supervision session. This review helps the supervisee in several ways. First, the supervisee's anxiety is lowered. The tape review usually shows that the session was not as bad as the supervisee feared. Also, the supervisee has some confidence during the supervision session by being able to point out good and bad points to the supervisor. Supervisors may request that supervisees develop questions or topics for examination, thereby making the supervisee assume considerable responsibility for the supervision session. Sometimes a supervisor will ask that the supervisee select only a few segments of the tape to be played and discussed during supervision. Supervisors may wish to give supervisees a rating form or checklist that the supervisee uses to evaluate taped sessions. The rating sheet is reviewed along with a few selected tape segments during the supervision session. Sample rating sheets are found in Dimick and Krause (1975). Supervisees can consider the strengths and weaknesses of their skills and reflect on their conceptualization of the client in a nonthreatening environment with no pressure to react immediately as in supervision.

In addition to the supervisee listening to the tape before the supervision session, the supervisor can listen to the tape before the supervision session and note pertinent issues to be discussed and specific tape segments to be played during the session. The supervisor may also fill out a structured rating sheet in order to provide more specific feedback to the supervisee. An individual review of the tape by supervisors improves efficiency by eliminating tape segments that are of minor importance. An example of such a rating sheet is included in Dimick and Krause (1975).

Although either supervisor or supervisee can review the tape prior to the supervision sessions, using both procedures would be ideal. When both supervisor and supervisee individually review the tape before the supervision session, the content of the session will have been determined more thoughtfully, thus increasing the effectiveness of the session than if a tape is played with no prior review.

In addition to increased effectiveness, tape review aids the efficiency of the supervision session. When the tape has not been examined before the session, supervisor and supervisee must choose segments unsystematically, often missing important segments. When left to chance, long segments of the tape are often played with little interaction between supervisor and supervisee. By reviewing the tape before the session and determining segments to be examined, supervisor and supervisee have more time for discussing the tape.

A related point is that when an entire tape is not examined by the supervisor, either before or during supervision, supervisees are often disappointed and conclude that their supervisor cannot really know their skills. Similarly, supervisees frequently become frustrated when critiqued by a supervisor who has listened to only part of a clinical session and heard only the mistakes. Supervisors can improve relationships with supervisees and enhance their own credibility by listening to entire tapes.

Using Tapes in Supervision   Hamatz (1975) reported that he uses videotape in an innovative way that increases the efficiency of the supervisory session. As a supervisee conducts a clinical session, Hamatz watches the session on a closed-circuit television monitor while the session is also being videotaped. Through a second channel into the videotape recorder, Hamatz makes brief comments about the ongoing clinical session that are recorded on the videotape. Between the clinical session and the supervision session, the supervisee reviews the videotape, which includes the supervisor's comments. In the supervision session certain parts of the tape are reviewed in further detail or other issues stimulated by the tape are discussed.

Videotaping allows supervisors to focus specifically on the non-verbal behavior of the supervisee or of the client. In reviewing a particular segment a supervisor may turn down the audio portion of the videotape so that only the picture can be seen. Without the interference of the verbalizations, the nonverbal behavior of the interaction can be analyzed more clearly. In a similar way, a supervisor can blur the picture of a videotape allowing the sound to come through clearly. The supervisee can then focus more carefully on his or her voice tone or that of the client's.

Many supervisors use role-playing as an adjunct to reviewing a tape recording. After the supervisor and supervisee discuss a taped segment in which the supervisee used an inappropriate technique or an appropriate technique ineffectively, they can role-play an appropriate technique or role-play the technique to gain effectiveness. This sequence of seeing one's error, then rehearsing a new behavior is a powerful technique for learning.

Coaching

One of the most innovative supervisor techniques in recent years has been the direct intervention of a supervisor with a supervisee while a clinical session is in progress. The supervisor observes the clinical session through a one-way mirror or through a videotape recording system and at particular points the supervisor speaks to the supervisee by telephone, by electronic bug in the ear, by having the supervisee leave the room, or by entering the room directly. Following the brief interaction with the supervisor, the supervisee returns to work with the client. Coaching gives the supervisor the opportunity to correct errors and strengthen conceptualizations exactly when needed. As a result, the supervisee applies the learnings immediately. Because of the brief nature of the interaction between supervisor and supervisee, interventions by the supervisor are usually a specific observation and evaluation followed by a concrete suggestion. Therefore, this supervisory technique is particularly suited to and primarily used within the Skill Development model of supervision. Montalvo (1973), Birchler (1975), and Hare-Mustin (1976) described their use of coaching (termed *live* supervision) in helping therapists to learn techniques of structural family therapy.

One specific method of coaching, the electronic bug in the ear (Boylston & Tuma, 1972, Tentoni & Robb, 1977), is particularly creative. In this method the supervisor observes the clinical session and speaks to the supervisee through an audio receiver located in the supervisee's ear. This procedure allows the supervisor to make a corrective suggestion to the supervisee in a less obtrusive way than calling in via the telephone or having the supervisee leave the room. Of course, when a powerful intervention is needed, such as entering the room with the clinician, the supervisor should use it. Positive results have been reported on the use of coaching (Liddle & Smith, 1977, 1978); however, a disadvantage is that the supervisor is forced to make a very brief comment or suggestion to the super-'visee with little or no explanation, and the supervisee has little opportunity but to carry out the suggestion.

A major criticism of coaching is that the supervisor will force the supervisee into a dependent relationship with the supervisor. Supposedly, the supervisee will become a skilled imitator of the supervisor but will not be able to integrate techniques into a more authentic relationship or be creative with new techniques that are developed. The counter-argument is that a supervisor does not nec-essarily force a supervisee to carry out the will of the supervisor but can help the supervisee who is at an impasse with a client and/ or is in the beginning stages of training and needs skills. Further-more, supervisee dependence is apparently quite pervasive at the beginning of supervision but changes as a supervisee develops knowledge and skills (Nelson, 1978). This development suggests that supervisory techniques (such as coaching) that build skills ef-ficiently may help supervisees to become independent more quickly because their confidence increases. Exploratory research by Liddle, Tannenbaum and Maloy (1980) gives initial support for this position.

One further criticism of coaching is that it interferes with the clinician-client relationship thought to be sacrosanct in many the-oretical orientations. The response of those using coaching is that the relationship can not only stand the interruption but also profit from it because the client has an understanding clinician in the room and a concerned supervisor monitoring the interaction. Re-search on the reactions of clients to coaching would be helpful to guide the use of this technique.

Overall, coaching is a highly intrusive technique that may cause some strong reactions among supervisees although large gains in learning may also be achieved. Any form of coaching will be aided by the sequence described earlier of planning for the therapy session by supervisor and supervisee, note-taking during the therapy session by supervisor, and a discussion between su-pervisor and supervisee following the therapy session. This creative supervisory technique, although expensive because of the high costs of observation rooms or television monitoring equipment, is worthy of consideration by supervisors.

Co-therapy

Several formats exist for using co-therapy as a method of supervision. Co-therapy as a supervisory technique usually consists of a supervisor and supervisee who work as a pair with a group or family from the beginning to the end of the clinical process. The form discussed early in the literature (Anker & Duffey, 1958) posits a senior clinician working with a less-experienced person. The senior clinician functions as a supervisor and the junior clinician as the supervisee. McGee (1968) and Coché (1977) agree that this format has distinct advantages and disadvantages. On one hand the supervisor can model precisely the professional behavior that the supervisee is supposed to learn (Silverman & Quinn, 1974) and can serve as an emotional support for a novice clinician. On the other hand, according to McGee (1968) "the presence of a skilled senior co-therapist has an anxiety-arousing and emotionally inhibiting effect on the supervisee" (p. 179). The fears of the supervisee of being evaluated by the supervisor or of disappointing the supervisor may inhibit the supervisee's clinical behavior. In general, this form of co-therapy supervision is suggested for advanced clinicians and should be preceded by other forms of co-therapy supervision (Grossman & Karmol, 1973).

In another form of co-therapy supervision a team of co-therapists of equivalent experience and training are jointly supervised by a third person who is more skilled in clinical work (Tucker et al., 1976). For example, in a university setting, two students would be paired as co-therapists and would be supervised by a faculty member. The supervisor reviews the work of the two supervisees by such means as their verbal report, direct observation through a one-way mirror, or tape recordings. Using two supervisees of equal training removes the hierarchy present in a supervisee-supervisor dyad. Coché (1977) stated, "The two students usually become very supportive of each other, which allows them to be creative and take risks" (p. 242). The development of the complex relationship between co-therapists changes, however, during the course of supervision. As Tucker and Liddle (1978) stated, "A developmental or evolutionary quality to the co-therapy relationships could be discerned as the training year progressed. At the outset, most trainee-trainee co-therapy relationships were characterized by caring and concern about each other, yet these relationships had elements of uncertainty and competitiveness" (p. 19). Clearly, supervisory techniques must be considered in a developmental framework if their effectiveness is to be accurately assessed.

As with other supervisory techniques each clinical session should be preceded by a planning session and followed by a discussion session between the co-clinicians. The discussion session is particularly important for co-therapists and has been thoroughly described by Tucker et al. (1976) who observed co-therapist supervisees through a one-way mirror. The first goal of the supervision session immediately following a therapy session was "to elicit the reactions of the co-therapists to each other and to the session" (Tucker et al., 1976, p. 270). The purpose of this goal is to solve any problems that occur as a result of the co-therapists' relationships with each other. Once the relationship between co-therapists is functional, learning and effective practice can be pursued.

The effectiveness of co-therapy as a supervisory technique is based on the effectiveness of co-therapy as a therapeutic approach. Coché (1977) thoroughly reviews the research on co-therapy and suggests that the advantages include: modeling for the clients, client problems surface quickly, less content is missed, and opportunities for creative interventions are facilitated. Authors reported by Coché (1977) mention several disadvantages including increased complexity of interaction, possibility of problems between leaders, and expense. Although some reservations have been expressed about co-therapy per se (Gans, 1962; McLennan, 1965), most authors concur that co-therapy is a valuable supervisory technique (McGee, 1968; McGee & Schuman, 1970).

Group Work

Group supervision is a technique in which a supervisor works with several supervisees at the same time. Several formats for conducting group supervision are available, each appropriate to the goals of particular models of supervision. In the Skill Development model the case conference and group discussion formats are used most frequently. Other formats will be discussed in Chapters 4 and 5.

The case conference consists of a meeting of supervisees of various levels of training and experience with a supervisor in which a supervisee presents a comprehensive description of a particular client, group, or family. Information obtained from tests, other professionals, medical records, etc. is presented. The supervisee also describes the course of therapy thus far, which usually includes an initial case conceptualization, goals, the approach, significant techniques used, and an estimation of their effects. After this presentation, the other supervisees and the supervisor ask questions and give suggestions that will help the supervisee to gain a clearer conceptualization of the client and to acquire new techniques. The group modality allows for many creative ideas to be generated and discussed. The supervisor participates by offering suggestions and questions yet also must direct the group as would a seminar insructor.

The group discussion is more informally structured than the case conference. In the group discussion, supervisees meet without designating a member to make a formal presentation. The supervisees share their ideas about their clients and receive suggestions from other supervisees in a loosely structured manner. A variety of topics can be discussed and are described by Liddle (1979).

Other supervisory techniques may be used as an adjunct to the case conference or the group discussion. Such techniques include role-playing, tape recordings, and observation. Observation was used by Tucker et al. (1976) and Tucker and Liddle (1978) who had a group of eight supervisees view a pair of supervisees through a one-way mirror. Immediately after the family therapy session, the three supervisors and all ten supervisees met and discussed the session that had been viewed. The goals of this case conference were: "a) to elicit reactions of the co-therapists to each other, b) to analyze observed family dynamics as a group, c) to make generalizations about the observed family and family therapy in general, d) to plan for future sessions with the family, and e) to express and discuss reactions to and feelings about the supervision" (Tucker et al., 1976, p. 270). These goals illustrate the type of goals that groups can accomplish with the case conference or group discussion techniques within the framework of the Skill Development model of supervision.

Group supervision, when used to accomplish the goals of the Skill Development model, has certain strengths and weaknesses. Supervisees benefit from their exposure to a wider variety of clients than is contained in their own case load. Consequently, their range of conceptual references and examples of client behavior is expanded. Furthermore, a variety of techniques and treatment strategies are generated from which an individual supervisee can choose. Also, the opportunity exists for feedback from a variety of points of view directed toward a particular supervisee's clinical efforts. When the group is the only mode of supervision, however, each supervisee gets little individual attention. Furthermore, the group may suffer as a result of personality clashes, reluctant members, or other group phenomena such as those that have weakened the impact of group therapy (Yalom, 1975). Many of the principles for conducting effective group therapy and effective classroom learning can be applied to group supervision in the Skill Development model of supervision.

Peers

Peer supervision is the mutual interaction between a pair or among a group of clinicians with no designated supervisor present. The peers could be students or clinicians on the job who are similar in skills, training, or organizational position. Peers can be instructed by a supervisor or decide by themselves to focus on skill acquisition (Hare & Frankena, 1972; Winstead et al., 1974; Seligman, 1978) or on personal growth (Allen, 1976) or some of both (Wagner & Smith, 1979).

A key assumption underlying peer supervision is that when supervisees interact without a supervisor a greater degree of mutual trust will be established than if a supervisor is present. This assumption is based on the notion that people who are similar and pose no threat of evaluation to each other will establish a greater degree of trust than those who are dissimilar, such as a supervisor and supervisees. Research is often done, however, where advanced students are paired with beginning students (Seligman, 1978) and so dissimilarity exists from the outset, thus making peer a misnomer. Davis and Arvey (1978) did not use the term peer when they used doctoral students, under the supervision of a faculty member, to supervise masters-level students in psychology. In this way the masters-level students perhaps felt less threat from a doctoral student than from a supervisor but may also have felt some respect for the doctoral student's advanced position and skills. Kendall (1972) and Wagner and Smith (1979) took a step to increase the effectiveness of peer interaction by training students to play the role of a supervisor; however, this differentiation in roles is likely to have added the evaluative dimension as in all supervisor-supervisee exchanges.

Research on groups of peers (Todd & Pine, 1968; Hare & Frankena, 1972; Winstead et al., 1974; Allen, 1976) has shown that similarity of training and years of experience among the members are often outweighed by dissimilarity of attitudes and differences in skills thus resulting in hierarchy among members and clearly perceived roles of supervisor and supervisee. The position supported in this volume is that peers can help each other to achieve skill development as shown by Seligman (1978) and other goals associated with other models of supervision; however, differences among pairs or groups of supervisees always will be perceived immediately following minimal interaction and these perceptions may or may not be helpful. Mutual trust is important but, as Mueller and Kell (1972) contend, evaluation apprehension exists in all relationships. Whether trust is higher and evaluation fears lower among peer supervisors than supervisor-supervisee dyads is unproved. Furthermore, whether confidence regarding evaluation is more important than respect for and confidence in a supervisor's superior skill remains to be explored. Peer supervision, like other supervisory techniques, should be applied judiciously and in combination with other techniques as part of an overall supervisory experience.

APPLICATION OF THE SKILL DEVELOPMENT MODEL

The Skill Development model of supervision is used with students and clinicians in agencies at all levels of training and experience. Although each supervisor has a particular style of conducting supervision there are certain parameters and guidelines to follow regarding teaching approach, as well as when and with whom the model should be applied. Following the discussion of the application of the model, an evaluation of the model will be presented that focuses on issues including dependency of the supervisee on the supervisor, disruptiveness of certain techniques, and the objectivity and efficiency of the model.

Guidelines

A key point in the Skill Development model of supervision occurs when the supervisor points out behaviors of the supervisee that were inappropriate, improperly timed, or ineffective. At this point the supervisor chooses either a direct or indirect instructional approach. That is, the supervisor chooses between informing the supervisee of what should have been done (direct instruction) or examining the supervisee's intentions for the technique used and the outcome of the technique with the client (indirect instruction). By the direct instruction approach the supervisor gives evaluative reactions to specific supervisee techniques with clients and offers suggestions of what to do differently in order to be more effective. The indirect approach includes rewarding positive behaviors, ignoring ineffective behavior, and mutually generating alternative techniques rather than specifying them. For example, a supervisor may directly instruct the supervisee by evaluating the supervisee's behavior using terms as good, bad, appropriate, or inappropriate. In this instance the supervisor and not the supervisee has applied the criteria for effective and ineffective clinical practice to the supervisee's work. Another example of the direct instructional approach is the supervisor's suggesting strategies or techniques for the supervisee to implement. The notion in this case is that the supervisor's approach or technique would have been more effective than that used by the supervisee or, if the supervisor mentions a strategy for future use, that this strategy will be more effective than one that might be selected by the supervisee.

A supervisor using the indirect instructional approach examines the supervisee's technique in terms of the client's response and whether this response was desirable according to the goals for the clinical session. In this way the criteria for the effective supervisee behavior is based on the client's response, not the supervisor's opinion. When a different technique is appropriate for the supervisee, a supervisor could elicit from the supervisee suggestions for alternate techniques and then discuss the pros and cons of each alternative. The supervisor might add alternatives not mentioned by the supervisee. Next, the supervisor helps the supervisee choose the technique that seems most likely to be successful with the client and, equally important, one that is consistent with the supervisee's theory of clinical practice and behavior change. If a supervisee does not believe that a particular technique is appropriate or does not adhere to the philosophy on which the technique is based, then using the technique will have limited effectiveness. By helping the supervisee to evaluate and choose techniques, the supervisor is communicating confidence in the supervisee's clinical ability, thus encouraging the supervisee to take a major role in the learning process.

Both approaches are valuable and may have differential effects depending on the preferred learning styles of supervisees. Worthington and Roehlke (1979) surveyed supervisor's behaviors according to their relationship to the perceptions of supervisor competence, satisfaction with supervision and improved counseling as perceived by beginning supervisees. One cluster of behaviors was related to giving direct instruction to supervisees regarding skills, (direct approach), yet another cluster was related to encouraging supervisees to develop their own counseling style (indirect approach). The effectiveness of the direct and indirect instructional approach with supervisees at different levels of development is one particular area that needs investigation.

Another guideline for supervisors who apply the Skill Development model is to emphasize the goals of both case conceptualization and skill acquisition. Some supervisors emphasize one of these goals to the exclusion of the other, sometimes at the request of the supervisee who does not value both goals equally. A typical sequence would be for a supervisor to help a supervisee conceptualize a case and then select appropriate techniques. If the supervisee conceptualized a case quickly, then more time could be spent on selecting an approach or practicing a technique. An effective ratio of time spent on case conceptualization and skill development would vary with each supervisee.

Techniques of the supervisor have been separated in this volume but are often used in combination with each other, which may produce greater gains in supervisee learning. For example, a videotape of a supervisee's session with a client may be reviewed by supervisee and supervisor and by supervisee and a peer. Or a supervisor may observe a therapy session of the supervisee with other supervisees and other supervisors then discuss the session with everyone. The combinations of techniques offer a wide range to creative supervisors although techniques should not be an end in and of themselves and should not be used indiscriminately.

Supervisors using these many techniques should consider several guidelines when applying any one or a combination of techniques. One guideline is to determine which technique would be most appropriate for supervisees with certain intellectual characteristics. Berengarten (1957) described the major learning patterns of social work students as either 1) doing, 2) experimental-empathic, or 3) intellectual-empathic. The "doer" learns best from specific directions regarding concrete tasks. This person is highly motivated by praise gained from teachers and supervisors regarding the successful completion of tasks. The experimental-empathic learner tries out hunches and relies on the results of intuitively proceeding with tasks that seem to be appropriate. The intellectual-empathic learner relies on deliberate plans that are carefully thought-out before any action is taken. Once an initial conceptualization is made, actions will follow with little difficulty. Rosenthal (1977) examined more specifically the effects of learning style and conceptual level of supervisees on the learning of clinical skills. His results indicated that the effectiveness of the method of teaching a clinical skill (confrontation) was dependent upon the conceptual level (high or low) of the supervisee. Kimberlin and Friesen (1977) suggested that level of cognitive complexity of the supervisee affects the impact of videotape or film, audiotape, or written examples used to convey therapeutic skills. Tinsley and Tinsley (1977) found a correlation between supervisee needs, interests, and abilities and the performance of students in training programs. Research in this important area has just begun and so supervisors must continue to rely on intuition until a clear direction is indicated.

A further guideline for effective supervision is for supervisors to use techniques that would not only be understood by supervisees (conceptual level) but also would be nonthreatening (emotional pattern). Of course, some anxiety will be created by any supervisory technique or discussion; but, most supervisors would agree that some techniques produce more anxiety than others. Also, some supervisees become anxious more quickly and to a greater extent than others. The strategy advocated here is to sequence supervisory techniques beginning with low-anxiety techniques and moving later to techniques of a more threatening nature. For example, a supervisor could start with self-report by the supervisee and later move to role-playing, followed by either sitting-in or observation, and then tape review. Although this sequence may not be ideal for all supervisees, the pattern advocated in this volume is for supervisees to become confident about verbally describing their work, which in turn allows them to face the more difficult task of examining their actual work with a client in the company of a supervisor.

A final area of application of the Skill Development model is when the model should be applied in terms of the level of a person's professional development. The differences between beginning and advanced supervisees is an area that has been examined only recently in psychology and psychiatry. It is generally believed that beginning supervisees in formal training programs want to know what to do and how to do it (Nelson, 1978; Worthington & Roehlke, 1979). Whether the beginning supervisee is a masters degree student or an advanced psychiatric resident (Schowalter & Pruett, 1975), the request for advice, structure, and direction is made. Apparently, supervisors can help beginning supervisees most by direct instruction rather than by an approach that focuses less clearly on what a supervisee should do with clients (Payne & Gralinski, 1968; Birk, 1972; Payne, Weiss, & Kapp, 1972; Payne, Winter, & Bell, 1972).

As described by Hogan (1964) and Clark (1965), however, supervision does not remain static; it changes as the process continues. "As counselors become more experienced," according to Worthington and Roehlke, "they may come to value more highly receiving feedback about their counseling behaviors within an unstructured relationship. They may also come to value less being taught new counseling behaviors within a structured relationship" (1979, p. 71). Supervisors must be sensitive to the supervisee's development, which may suggest new behavior by the supervisor using the Skill Development model.

Evaluation

The Skill Development model is a highly effective and frequently used model of supervision with students in training programs and clinicians on the job. The effectiveness and frequency of use is attributable, in part, to the focus on observable behavior of the client and supervisee. The supervisor using this model can establish a list of areas or skills with the supervisee on which the supervisee will become knowledgeable and proficient (Tomm & Wright, 1979). This knowledge and proficiency can be measured in terms of actual supervisee behavior with clients. Measurement of the effectiveness of supervision according to demonstrated supervisee proficiency with clients is a step recommended by Hansen, Pound, and Petro (1976) in their five-year review of supervision research in psychology.

Because the Skill Development model is relatively objective, it also helps therapy become more objective. When supervision is seen as case conceptualization resulting in specific goals and skills, therapy becomes more of a science than an art. Making therapy more objective reduces anxiety of supervisees because they are evaluated in terms of what they do with clients, not who they are as people. Reducing anxiety to a moderate level will help supervisees learn more efficiently. To be sure, supervisees become anxious about evaluation of their conceptualizations and skills, but making a mistake because of a thought or a skill produces less anxiety than being judged deficient because of a personality characteristic.

Not only is the Skill Development model effective, but it also is efficient. Faculty supervisors have a limited amount of time in which to establish minimum competence in their students. Agency supervisors are responsible to the clients and to the agency administrators for ensuring that supervisees provide an acceptable quality of service. Of course, certain supervisory techniques such as audiotape and videotape review or observation require expensive equipment and physical facilities. Furthermore, techniques such as sitting-in, observation, and co-therapy require valuable supervisory time and are costly. If, however, the overall goal is to have supervisees attain initial competence in conceptualization or particular clinical techniques, the Skill Development model is best suited for this purpose. Original research in psychology by Cormier, Hackney, & Segrist (1974), Toukmanian and Rennie (1975), and

Ivey (1978) and reviews of research by Hansen and Warner (1971), Matarazzo (1978), and Hansen et al. (1976) strongly support the effectiveness and efficiency of the Skill Development model.

The overall emphasis in the Skill Development model on the supervisee as learner of a craft is particularly helpful for beginning clinicians both in training at a university and on the job. In the fields of psychiatry and psychology, more so than in social work, bachelors degree programs consist mostly of didactic courses. Students entering advanced training have acquired few skills in a formal manner and so their instructors strongly emphasize skill acquisition during these advanced training programs (Hart, 1979). Because faculty in these programs tend to emphasize the acquisition of clinical knowledge and skills more than, for example, the enhancement of the student as a person, it is likely that the Skill Development model is applied more often than other models during practicum, field work, or residence.

The Skill Development model is also used frequently in agencies with professionals who have little prior experience. Supervisors can quickly allay supervisee anxiety by focusing on skills and conceptualizations of clients. Apparently, case conceptualization is stressed more frequently than skill acquisition, perhaps because supervisors in agencies assume that beginning workers have the necessary skills once case conceptualizations are established.

One of the most significant issues in all models of supervision is the usefulness of supervisory techniques that intervene in the clinician-client interaction, such as sitting-in or coaching. Some authors (Cooper, 1975) believe that techniques such as audiotaping or videotaping threaten the client and thereby disrupt the therapeutic process between clinician and client. Abroms (1977) and Melchiode (1977) contend that information gained from techniques other than supervisee self-report lessen the importance of the supervisee's perceptions. In other words, through observation, etc., the supervisor will rely more on his or her own perceptions of the clinical session than on the perception of the supervisee, thereby undermining the supervisor-supervisee relationship.

A closely related contention emphasizes that supervisees tend to bias and distort reality through their self-report of a clinical session (Fleming & Benedek, 1966; Ekstein & Wallerstein, 1972). Consequently, supervisors are urged to become aware of these biases and distortions and to point them out to the supervisee, thereby enhancing the supervisees' "clinical judgment." The point is made that these biases will not be displayed when a direct observation by the supervisor is made.

The usual justification for the supervisors' observing a therapy session is that the supervisor can then view all details of the session, not just the details brought up by the supervisee, and that the more information gathered, the better the service to the client and to the supervisee. A study by Stein et al. (1975) showed that, indeed, supervisors had a different perception of patients observed directly than patients described wholly by their supervisees. These authors advise that, "Direct observation of the patient by the supervisor in the initial interview is an important factor in the accuracy of patient evaluation. This allows the supervisor to guide the resident in formulating an appropriate treatment plan, which is important for both improved training and better patient care" (Stein et al., 1975, p. 268). It is not that the supervisee's points are wrong and the supervisor's points are right but that their perceptions are different and both have value. Furthermore, a supervisor's independent observation of the supervisee's performance through observation, taping, or sitting-in does not necessarily mean that the supervisor-supervisee relationship will deteriorate, just that a potential conflict may exist between them, and if so, the resolution may lead to negative or positive results.

The entire issue of supervisory interventions rests, to some extent, on the supervisor's beliefs about conflicts. Supervisors range from those who believe that conflict on many issues is inevitable and discussion of conflict when it occurs can be positive, to those who believe that all conflict is negative and should be avoided through the use of nonthreatening supervisory techniques. Active supervisory techniques, indeed, are more intrusive than self-report, and intrusions cause more rapid change. Initial research findings by Liddle, Tannenbaum, and Maloy (1980) show that coaching, for example, is not detrimental to the therapeutic and supervisory processes and is often quite helpful to both. Supervision is viewed in this volume as the management of changes in the supervisee toward ideal professional behavior. Conflicts that arise are seen here as valuable because the issues underlying them may never have surfaced without the impetus from an intrusive supervisory technique. Supervisees show biases in many ways regardless of the supervisory technique implemented and those biases can be examined in the discussion between supervisor and supervisee at any time, not just following a self-report of the supervisee about a client. Active supervisory techniques will involve obtaining new data for the supervisor, and certainly will create strains on the supervisory relationship; but, supervisory techniques will not be unduly disruptive if the relationship is strong enough.

A closely related criticism of the Skill Development model is that the supervisor as expert and the supervisee as novice contributes to supervisee dependence on the supervisor. The supervisee will come to rely on the supervisor for answers and will be relatively unable to generate answers without the supervisor. Similarly, supervisees may become dependent on supervisors for validation of their competence. These charges have not been explored in a research format but anecdotal reports suggest that supervisee dependence, like client dependence, is a possibility in some supervisee-supervisor relationships. The key element may not be the goal of the model, for example, skill development, but the encouragement, albeit subtle, of the supervisee to become dependent. Some dependence is probably inevitable among most beginning supervisees and is probably related to the supervisee's identification with the supervisor. The supervisor who encourages dependence throughout supervision, however, by discouraging the supervisee from taking risks or making independent decisions does the supervisee a disservice. Such behavior, it is believed, is not necessarily characteristic of the Skill Development model.

The Skill Development model of supervision, through a variety of techniques and technology, has become a widely used model. The relative effectiveness of specific techniques with certain supervisees remains to be determined. Research is particularly needed with supervisees of various levels of emotional and intellectual characteristics. A comparison of beginning and advanced supervisees would be particularly useful in terms of which techniques are most effective for supervisees at various developmental levels. Furthermore, research needs to focus less on comparison of several techniques (or several models) with a group of heterogeneous supervisees and more on the effectiveness of a single technique (or a single model) on various distinct homogeneous groups of supervisees. Overall, the Skill Development model has made great strides in helping supervisees gain initial therapeutic competence.

SUMMARY

In this chapter the Skill Development model of supervision is described according to the two goals of case conceptualization and skill acquisition. The Skill Development model has been shown to be an effective and efficient way of helping supervisees to understand client behavior and to gain clinical skills. Some of the factors that encourage the use of this model include the variety of available supervisory techniques, the demand for this approach by beginning supervisees, and the efficiency of this model in terms of time. The Skill Development model is clearly a primary model of supervision; however, much research is needed in order to learn how the model can be used with intermediate and advanced supervisees and with supervisees of various levels of emotional and intellectual characteristics.

Chapter 4

Personal Growth Model

RATIONALE FOR THE MODEL

Most supervisors and supervisees would probably agree that effective clinicians need to be insightful and emotionally sensitive if they are to be maximally effective with their clients. Considerable disagreement exists, however, as to the responsibility of the university or the agency to promote these qualities through supervision. Even those faculty members or agency staff members who believe that insight and sensitivity should be promoted through supervision find few guidelines to follow so that personal growth does not become therapy. In this chapter the issue of supervision as personal growth or therapy is explored so that supervisors can see the rationale for growth activities in their supervision of clinicians.

From psychiatry and particularly psychoanalysis several reviews of literature on supervision (DeBell, 1963; Schlessinger, 1966) document the responsibility of the supervisor to help the supervisee "to achieve an awareness of his own character problems which may interefere with the establishment and maintenance of a therapeutic relationship" (Wolberg, 1951, p. 150). Wolberg represents the predominant position in psychiatry; that is, students will experience certain emotions toward patients, and this experiencing is termed *countertransference*. Countertransference, according to Fleming (1953), means "the behavior of the therapist as it is motivated by unconscious and inappropriate reactions to his patent stemming from confused identification of his relationship to the patient with his relationship to other persons in this past" (p. 161). The "character problems" mentioned by Wolberg and the "confused identification" identified by Fleming support the need for an approach that is aimed at remediation rather than enhancement. The assumption is that supervisees have problems or unresolved conflicts that should be eliminated through therapy conducted concurrently with supervision or therapy conducted during supervision.

Some authors (Ferber, 1972; Kaslow, 1977; Guldner, 1978) strongly recommend or require that all supervisees engage in personal therapy, separate from supervision, as a part of their training program. Educators and supervisors who support this position assume that every supervisee has deficits to remedy or weaknesses to improve but that these problems may not be the ones suggested by authors such as Wolberg and Fleming. Furthermore, a voluntary or required therapy experience is seen as helping supervisees to understand the position of being a client. Commonly, these supervisees engage in therapy for some predetermined period of time with someone other than their supervisor as therapist. An assumption of this position is that the clinicians who enter an agency or a training program have been carefully screened to allow only the most insightful and sensitive people into the agency or training program. Of course, no matter how careful the screening, some clinicians or students will have problems that need to be remediated, perhaps with long-term therapy.

Another position is that supervisees enter the training program or the agency with relatively high levels of personal development but will inevitably encounter situations that arouse thoughts and feelings not previously experienced. The supervisor who assumes responsibility for preparing the supervisee to meet these new thoughts and feelings may adopt an enhancement, rather than a problem-solving focus, and may help the supervisee to understand patterns of behavior and feelings the supervisee had never previously understood or identified. Of course, if a serious problem appears, the supervisor would refer the supervisee for therapy to be conducted concurrently with supervision or in lieu of supervision until the problem is resolved.

In this latter approach to supervision, focusing on personal thoughts and feelings may be confused with the focusing on personal thoughts and feelings that occurs in therapy. For this reason it is important to compare and contrast therapy with personal growth activities in supervision. In supervision, therapy, and good interpersonal relations, in general, the methods of establishing a relationship of trust, openness, and respect are quite similar. By appropriate self-disclosure of thoughts and feelings both past and present (Jourard, 1971) and by communication through empathic listening and nonjudgmental responses (Rogers, 1951, 1957), a dyad or a group can promote close interpersonal relationships. This parallel between supervision and therapy was pointed out by Pettes (1967), Melchiode (1977), and others who then concluded that such affective responses by a supervisor do not constitute a therapy session. A supervision session can *become* a therapy session, but affective responses that are designed to enhance the supervisory relationship are far from therapy.

A related point is that any behavior may have an unintended therapeutic effect given the right supervisee. That is, a supervisor's most casual remark or raising of an eyebrow could stimulate a supervisee to experience feelings and thoughts of which he or she was not previously aware. Even when a supervisor fully intends and attempts to be quite didactic in supervision, the supervisee will experience a combination of both cognitive and affective growth as concluded by Nash (1975). Such incidental or secondary reactions are possible in supervision just as in casual conversation among acquaintances, but the presence of such unplanned, albeit powerful, therapeutic events cannot define an entire supervision session or a series of sessions.

The biggest distinction between personal growth in supervision and therapy seems to be in the supervisor's response to supervisee statements regarding personal thoughts and feelings. On the one hand, Gitelson (1948), Ackerman (1953), Emch (1955), Ekstein and Wallerstein (1972), and Gaoni and Neumann (1974) believe that psychiatric supervisors should be alert to the neurotic patterns in supervisees and should confront such blind spots of the supervisee. For a supervisor to actively interpret the meaning of a particular supervisee's comment in the analytical sense would be therapy. Grotjahn (1955) and Searles (1955) urge supervisors to be cautious in judging their supervisee's problems, however, and to leave such judgments to a therapist. Their thesis is supported by Spiegel and Grunebaum (1977) who describe the anger of psychiatric residents toward supervisors who point out unresolved problems and suggest therapy or analysis for the resident.

In a move away from therapy in the supervision session, Dewald (1969) advises supervisors to help supervisees engage in "self-analysis." Supervisors are urged to use the approach of "avoidance of too-active or complete interpretations that might foster passivity in the student in regard to self-analysis, tolerance toward the existence of countertransference in the student, helping the student to see his or her countertransference and counterreactions as data to be observed and used in the analytic process, questioning the student about his personal feeling or associations to the patient's material, and indicating general patterns of countertransference or predicting possible occurrence" (Dewald, 1969, p. 119). Ekstein and Wallerstein (1972) agree that the feelings and attitudes of the supervisee should be discussed but without references to unresolved conflicts or a neurotic basis for the feelings and attitudes.

Searles (1955) and Mueller and Kell (1972) move still farther from therapy by describing how a supervisor should use the feelings of the supervisee as data that describe the relationship between the supervisee and client. For example, a supervisee who expresses anger toward a particular client who was consistently late for appointments would be directed to examine the possibility that the client may be communicating some message to the supervisee through the lateness. The supervisor helps the supervisee examine the relationship with the client and notes similarities and differences between their relationship and client's (or supervisee's) relationships with others who are late. A summary of the various positions is that when a supervisor shifts from *what* the supervisee thought and felt to *why or what caused* the ideas and feelings to occur, the process also shifts from supervision to therapy.

The primary justification for increasing the level of supervisee personal growth comes from the fact that strong feelings and thoughts about self do arise during one's clinical practice whether in a training program or an agency. Two main reasons exist for the arousal of strong feelings and thoughts among supervisees. In work settings where intense psychotherapy is conducted and in programs where students are trained to conduct such therapy, therapists often work with very psychologically disturbed clients. These clients may also discuss subjects that may be unusual or shocking to the therapist such as drug abuse, violence, or incest. The shocked therapist becomes less effective. The supervisor should aid the therapist in coping with emotional reactions to such cases in order to help the therapist be more secure, which eventually allows the therapist to be more effective.

A second reason for arousal of powerful thoughts and feelings in therapists is that intense psychotherapy evokes the expression of strong emotional responses by clients. Client expression of feeling can in turn provoke strong feelings and thoughts within therapists that can decrease their effectiveness. Supervisors should prepare supervisees for these thoughts and feelings in order to cope with them more effectively. These feelings and thoughts can be ignored by the supervisor who may hope that the supervisee explores them outside supervision or they can be brought into supervision as a basis for discussion. The contention of the Personal Growth model is that such discussion will improve the interpersonal functioning of the supervisee thus resulting in more effective clinical behavior with clients. Clearly, the supervisee's emotional and cognitive reactions to clients can have an effect on one's therapeutic outcome, but how does a supervisor determine whether to approach such personal issues with the supervisee?

Several guidelines emerge from the literature concerning a supervisor's approach to a supervisee's personal issues. One guideline is for the supervisor to determine the degree to which the supervisee's professional functioning with the client is impaired. The supervisor assesses the client's reactions over time to determine if the supervisee's feelings or attitudes negatively affect the client. If a negative effect is shown, then the supervisee's attitudes and feelings are examined during supervision. This guideline is based on the view described earlier that supervisees will inevitably have unresolved emotional conflicts that will surface during therapy with clients and should be resolved during a supervision process that is, or approximates, therapy. A cue for the supervisor, according to Chessick (1971), is the anxiety level of the supervisee. He stated, "The anxiety level [of the supervisee] is the crucial factor in determining to what extent the supervisor should be purely didactic and to what extent he should begin to approach unconscious process in the resident that are interfering with his work with patients" (Chessick, 1971, p. 276). The intent of supervision, according to Chessick, is analogous to the intent of therapy in that the supervisor should uncover the problems of the supervisee when the supervisee's anxiety rises to a level that suggests remediation is needed.

A second guideline for approaching supervisees' personal thoughts and feelings is that all of these personal reactions affect supervisees' interpersonal functioning with both clients and others in their lives. Supervisors who believe that supervisees should be aware of the effects of their thoughts and feelings upon their interpersonal relations will focus on this issue with the supervisee. These supervisors will not wait for signs that clients are not progressing or that supervisees are highly anxious. These supervisors believe in promoting the growth of the supervisee, not in resolving personal problems of the supervisee through supervision. The Personal Growth model is an important method for promoting supervisee growth.

DESCRIPTION OF THE MODEL

The Personal Growth model, like other models of supervision, is based on an effective relationship between supervisor and supervisee. Conant (1976) and Nash (1975) surveyed supervisees and reported that unconditional positive regard and empathy of the supervisor are a large part of the supervisees' judgment of the quality of supervision received. Kadushin (1966) stated, "A positive relationship intensifies the impact of the supervisor's educational efforts. There is considerable empirical support for the contention that the nature of the relationship is a powerful variable in determining the supervisee's openness and receptivity to the supervisor's efforts to educate toward change" (p. 148). Brammer and Wassmer (1977) concluded that, "The facilitative characteristics which, when found in therapists, produce the greatest gains in clients seem identical or closely related to those characteristics which, when found in supervisors, produce the greatest gain in trainees" (p. 52).

Clearly, a positive supervisor-supervisee relationship is an important dimension in any model of supervision, but supervision in the Personal Growth model is more than a supportive relationship.

Reports of supervisees (Conant, 1976; Nash, 1975) show that the quality of the supervisory relationship, in terms of facilitative conditions expressed by the supervisor, has separate effects from those produced by the model of supervision. Because the quality of the relationship is separate from, albeit related to, the model of supervision, both aspects must be considered by researchers in their evaluation of supervision. Practically, supervisors who wish to bring about personal growth in supervisees must be aware of the goals of the Personal Growth model that go beyond the supportive relationship that forms the basis of the interaction.

The purpose of the Personal Growth model of supervision is to increase insight and emotional sensitivity by examining the supervisee's interpersonal relationship patterns that exist beyond the special relationships with clients. The intent is not to resolve interpersonal problems the supervisee has—whether they are general problems or ones with a particular client—but to develop the supervisee's insight and emotional sensitivity. It is believed that all supervisees, especially those with minimal training or experience, can increase their skills in this area. Words such as "insight" and "emotional sensitivity" were chosen by Rogers (1957), Arbuckle (1963), Patterson (1964), Altucher (1967) and others to label the goals of the Personal Growth model. Because these authors have a phenomenological view toward therapy such terms are likely to connote a phenomenological view of supervision. Indeed, supervisors with other orientations to therapy may have avoided the Personal Growth model of supervision because of these phenomenological connotations. The Personal Growth model of supervision, although certainly based on phenomenological principles, is not restricted to using the phenomenological approach in their clinical work. This model can be used by any supervisor who believes that a supervisee should develop personally as well as professionally even though supervisors may define personal development in widely differing terms. For example, a supervisee reported, "I've really learned how disappointed I get when other people don't do the things that I think are helpful for them. My disappointment shows and makes things worse." Supervisors who prefer the framework of transactional analysis might focus on the parent-adult-child ego positions assumed by the supervisee in personal relationships. Supervisors with a cognitive orientation (Mahoney, 1974; Beck, 1976) might direct the supervisee to examine thoughts about people in whom the supervisee has been disappointed. Increased sensitivity can be valued goals for supervisors with any orientation to therapy.

Developing Insight

The first goal of the personal growth model is to develop supervisee insight; that is, knowledge of existing patterns of interpersonal behavior not recognized at present by the supervisee. To increase insight a supervisor, for example, might assist the supervisee in a self-monitoring process to determine the supervisee's specific behaviors in a particular type of interpersonal situation. Mr. Bander, a supervisor in a drug treatment agency, assists Mr. Miller, a new clinician, in recording his reactions to people who are very emotionally detached because Mr. Miller will work with clients who display such behavior.

Defined as the knowledge or cognitive recognition of one's behavior patterns, the goal of achieving insight may be of interest primarily to supervisors whose therapeutic orientation is of a cognitive or behavioral nature. Supervisors whose therapeutic orientation includes the exploration of feelings will also spend some time on achieving insight as well as affective sensitivity. Of course, some supervisors have a strict psychodynamic view of therapy that precludes any examination of overt behavior, just as some supervisors have a strict behavioral orientation that prevents any emphasis on insight or affective sensitivity. Generally, supervisors are advised to develop both the cognitive and affective aspects of supervisees even though their model of therapy may focus more exclusively on either area.

Developing Affective Sensitivity

Affective sensitivity is the second goal of the Personal Growth model of supervision and is defined as the awareness of emotional reactions as they are experienced during interpersonal situations (Lister, 1966a). Sensitivity to one's emotions is viewed, by some, as a valuable source of data by which the relationships between supervisee and others can be assessed. To increase sensitivity a supervisor might, for example, discuss the supervisee's emotional reactions to people who are not punctual because the supervisee will encounter clients who are late. The supervisor would engage the supervisee in an introspective process using techniques that assist the supervisee in becoming aware of feelings that had not been identified previously.

These characteristics of the functional relationship between supervisor and supervisee, the hierarchy between the supervisor and supervisee, and the focus of the session differentiate the Personal Growth model from other models of supervision.

The functional relationship between supervisor and supervisee in the Personal Growth model is one of helper to helpee. The supervisor is clearly a person who assists the supervisee to examine interpersonal relationships in order to gain insight and/or affective sensitivity. The supervisor uses many clinical skills to help the supervisee in this self-examination process and somewhat resembles a clinician engaged in therapy. Correspondingly, the supervisee, like a willing client, accepts the position of receiving assistance in the self-examination process. The relationship is complementary in that both persons have different and mutually agreeable roles to play that fit or complement each other (Haley, 1963).

The hierarchical distance between supervisor and supervisee in the Personal Growth model ranges from high to moderate. The supervisor maintains some level of hierarchy in this range because of the duty to keep the supervisee focused on insight and/or affective sensitivity. Furthermore, an implication of this model is that the supervisee needs personal growth presumably more than the supervisor, thus establishing the supervisor as superior to the supervisee. This implied difference in the relative level of personal development between supervisor and supervisee contributes to the hierarchical distance between them. As described in Chapter 1, hierarchical distance is quite functional and appropriate for the roles of helper and helpee once supervisor and supervisee establish an acceptable distance.

The third characteristic, focus of the session, clearly distinguishes the Personal Growth model from other models of supervision. In the Personal Growth model, the focus of the session is on the supervisee's interpersonal relations with friends, relatives, or acquaintances. The focus is not on skills used with specific clients as in the Skill Development model or on a specific professional relationship with someone such as a current client, as in the Integration model. Furthermore, the focus in the Personal Growth model is less specific to the supervisee's work environment than the other two models. For example, a supervisee could explore ideas and feelings about relating to those who are older, of the opposite sex, or of a minority group as groups of people rather than as specific clients.

Focus in the Personal Growth model can be not only on groups or categories of people but also on specific individuals in the supervisee's life. If a supervisee begins to discuss relationships with a hostile client, then the supervisor expands the discussion to include relationships the supervisee has had with hostile people other than this particular client. This shift to nonprofessional relationships helps supervisees understand their typical behavior patterns and feelings, which will, in turn, have an impact on how they relate to many people, including clients.

CASE STUDY

This case study illustrates the typical responses of a supervisor using the Personal Growth model of supervision. The case is taken verbatim from *Styles of Supervision II*, a videotape developed by Hart (1976b) and the *Instructor Manual* for the videotape written by Hart et al. (1976b). The comments in the left-hand margin point out where the supervisor illustrates one of the factors of: 1) the functional relationship of the supervisor and supervisee, 2) the hierarchical relationship between supervisor and supervisee, and 3) the focus of the session.

Comments	Supervisor-Supervisee Interaction

	Supervisee:
	    Hi, Mel.
	Supervisor:
	    Hi, Frank, how are you?
	Supervisee:
	    Oh, pretty good.
	Supervisor:
	    How've you been?
	Supervisee:
	    Okay, really, I don't know, I have something I'd like to talk to you about.
	Supervisor:
	    Sure.
	Supervisee:
	    One of the cases, one of the clients I'm seeing. Refreshing your memory, her name is Janet, and I think I talked to you about her a few sessions ago. She's the one that's, uh, she's overdosed two or three times.
	Supervisor:
	    Oh, and she attempted suicide on a few occasions, did she not?

Comments	Supervisor-Supervisee Interaction
	Supervisee:
	Yes. She's cut her wrists. I don't know, this past weekend she just cut her wrists again and . . .
	Supervisor:
	So, this is the third attempt, or the fourth?
	Supervisee:
	I think it's the fourth now. And, I don't know, I'm just looking for a new direction to go in.
Supervisor shifts the focus from client data to the relationship between supervisee and client to make a transition from the Skill Development to the Personal Growth model.	**Supervisor:**
	Why don't you tell me something about the direction your relationship is taking now?
	Supervisee:
	Well, up to this point, we've been working on her walking out of the house if she was starting to get into an argument with her father. The other thing, I don't know, it was just talking about her feelings about her father, and digging it out on that.
	Supervisor:
	And where did that go?
	Supervisee:
	Well, I don't know. She really loves him, but she's very ambivalent about him. She loves him, but she hates him.
	Supervisor:
	What kinds of things were you *experiencing* in your dealings with Janet about her father?
	Supervisee:
	Well, I guess about a month ago I thought, you know, that we were really going to make progress because she came out with, well, she told me that she had an abortion about 2 years ago. And at that point, I gained a lot of insight where I thought that, well, possibly she can't express anger towards her father because she's hurt him so much.

Comments	Supervisor-Supervisee Interaction
	Supervisor: Did you allow that anger to come out in the session?
	Supervisee: Um, she wasn't, no, she didn't bring it up.
	Supervisor: Did you allow her to bring it up? Did you provide her with the format?
	Supervisee: Oh, I gave her enough time, yeah. I'm not, well, what do you mean by format?
Supervisor moves from the specific client to other clients as a way to get into the Personal Growth model.	Supervisor: I guess I'm kind of wondering what you would have done with the anger in that situation, how you, as a therapist, would have handled her anger, and what that might be saying about the way you *deal* with anger. Have you ever gotten angry with a client?
	Supervisee: Oh, yeah, yeah. I usually tell them. I tell them if I get mad at them.
	Supervisor: Do you tell them immediately, or do you think about it a great deal?
	Supervisee: I'd say I stop for a few seconds and I get it all together, how I'm going to put it out, and everything. It's not spontaneous.
	Supervisor: Okay, is it real?
	Supervisee: Oh, yeah, it's real, yeah.
Supervisor examines supervisee's typical expression of anger to people in general.	Supervisor: Is that characteristic of you when you are angry? How do you deal with anger?
	Supervisee: Myself?
	Supervisor: Yourself.
	Supervisee: Uh, I usually fly off into profanities, and stomp around.
	Supervisor: Just kind of let go?
	Supervisee: Oh, yeah.

Comments	Supervisor-Supervisee Interaction
	Supervisor:

Supervisor:
Um hum. Do you think it's appropriate to do that in a session?

Supervisee:
Uh, gee, no, I'd tend to hold it back.

Supervisor:
Okay, so then you're doing something, you're introducing something into that session that's bringing in the element of, maybe, unrealness, into the situation. You're not providing her with the real image of yourself.

Supervisee:
Yeah, I guess, yeah.

Supervisor gives an interpretation of the supervisee's behavior regarding expression of anger—the hierarchy between them is emphasized.

Supervisor:
And I guess what I'm looking at is maybe you're defending against something, that you're identifying yourself that you have pretty strong feelings about, and that, in turn, is inhibiting the session. You're not allowing her to get angry because maybe you're afraid of anger.

Supervisee:
That's quite possible. I guess if I was very . . . if I was a little bit more real, then she would be too, then, right?

Supervisor:
Um Hum. I guess I'm wondering, you know, how you would handle that anger and more importantly if you allowed it to come out, where would you go with it?

Supervisee:
Uh, well, if it came out of her, right?

Supervisor:
Yeah.

Supervisee:
I'd, you know, let it flow, in the direction it went. I'd tend to lay back and play the, uh, okay, I imagine she sees me as a father image.

Supervisor:
Are you comfortable with that image?

Supervisee:
Yeah, that's fine. As long as she doesn't throw things at me, you know.

Supervisor:
Um hum, I wonder if being that kind of a father figure, you're protecting in any

Comments	Supervisor-Supervisee Interaction
	way, you're protecting her, you're protecting yourself a little bit? Does that kind of make sense?
	Supervisee:
	Possibly, but I'm thinking along the lines of her reacting differently than she does at home, like maybe learn a new. . . .
	Supervisor:
	You're anticipating, then, the way she'll react.
	Supervisee:
	Yeah, yeah.
	Supervisor:
	Is that good?
	Supervisee:
	No, I guess not.
Supervisor acts as a helper and examines another aspect of the supervisee's personal behavior.	**Supervisor:**
	Do you anticipate every day, you know, the kind of things that might occur? Say, in your relationship with your father, you're living at home, can you anticipate the kind of things that might occur and react accordingly?
	Supervisee:
	Well, there is a certain range of behavior that I expect, but I mean, I can't, you know, actually you know. . . .
	Supervisor:
	Okay, I guess what I'm saying is that by anticipating her response in the session, maybe you're not allowing the session to flow in a realistic fashion, maybe you're cutting off some things that are a little difficult for you to handle.
	Supervisee:
	Um, yeah, yeah I think so, yeah.
	Supervisor:
	Okay, I guess in terms of exploring that, using yourself as an example, I would be concerned if it occurs with other clients.
	Supervisee:
	Hum. (Pause) I think you're right. I think I have, I'm thinking of two clients. There's one other girl I'm seeing, and she's been discussing her, I guess her love life.
	Supervisor:
	Okay, but there's a problem, again.

Comments	Supervisor-Supervisee Interaction
	Supervisee: Yeah.
Supervisor broadens the focus from a specific client to male and female clients as preparation to move to people in general.	**Supervisor:** We have two females. Could this occur in dealing with male clients?
	Supervisee: With males I think I take a different approach. **Supervisor:** Okay, then why? What is tempering your approach to males and females? **Supervisee:** I hadn't really thought about it before, but maybe I'm, gee, stereotyping.
Supervisor now broadens the focus to the supervisee's approach to people in general.	**Supervisor:** Well, okay. "Stereotyping" is a, it's an okay kind of word, but I'm wondering what that says about the way you relate to women and the way you relate to men. And as a counselor, do you relate differently, and what that says about your ability to help.
Supervisee responds with an insight that is a goal of this model and shows himself to be a helpee. Supervisor finds a pattern to the supervisee's reactions to women in general. Supervisor's interpretation shows the helper role and the large hierarchical distance between them.	**Supervisee:** Right. I guess I, I'd probably be able to help men, then. With women I guess I'm a little bit hung up about being open and real with them. **Supervisor:** Okay, so you're being a little bit defensive with women?
	Supervisee: Um hum. **Supervisor:** Okay, so there's Janet, and there's the other client, and I remember once before you mentioned another female you were working with, that you had an awful lot of problems, dealing with in terms of the behavioral model that you're coming from. Do you recall that?

Comments	Supervisor-Supervisee Interaction

	Supervisee:
	    Yes. Her name was Rose, yeah.
	Supervisor:
	    Now there was some resistance there,
	    too, wasn't there?
	Supervisee:
	    Yes, there was.
	Supervisor:
	    Okay. Are there any similarities
	    between the two cases we've discussed
	    and this, the third case?
	Supervisee:
	    Well. . . .

The supervisor in the above case used primarily the Personal Growth model. As described in Chapter 6, however, supervisors sometimes use more than one model within a particular session. The supervisor in this case example looked first for the supervisee's patterns of behavior with clients then changed the focus to relationships with nonclients. In addition, the supervisor used only the verbal self-report of the supervisee as a technique although other techniques could have been used, such as those described below.

TECHNIQUES

Any of the techniques described in Chapter 3 for the Skill Development model also could be applied within the Personal Growth model. Although some techniques lend themselves more to one model than another, such as coaching in the Skill Development model, creative supervisors should experiment with a variety of techniques regardless of an apparent relationship between a technique and a particular model. This experimentation may result in a combination of techniques that is particularly suited to the learning style of a specific supervisee or to several supervisees working with a specific agency or training institution.

Self-report

Verbal self-report by the supervisee of behavior, thoughts, and feelings was the technique used in the case study and is probably the technique used most frequently by supervisors using the Personal Growth model of supervision. The supervisor helps the supervisee to identify patterns of behavior or typical responses in order to help the supervisee gain insight and/or affective sensitivity.

Although the verbal self-report of a supervisee is used frequently within the Personal Growth model, a written self-report may also be used. Written self-reports consist of charts, surveys, questionnaires or other forms in which the supervisee writes out ideas and/or feelings in response to questions given by the supervisor. One form for use with supervisees is Are You Someone Who? found in *Values Clarification* (Simon, Howe, & Kirschenbaum, 1972). Other forms may be found in *A Handbook of Structured Experiences for Human Relations Training* (Pfeiffer & Jones, 1969), *Personalizing Education* (Howe & Howe, 1975), and *Self-directed Behavior* (Watson & Tharp, 1977). The supervisee's written responses become the material discussed between supervisor and supervisee. Typically, the supervisee completes the form outside of the supervision session and discusses the responses during the supervision session. In this way the supervisor establishes a clear structure for the supervisee and supervisor to follow and allows the supervisee to prepare for the supervision session.

Another written self-report technique is the log, which is also called the diary, journal, or autobiography. In this technique the supervisee keeps a written report on ideas and feelings that occur each day or week. The log may be completely unstructured or may follow guidelines as suggested by Sample Diaries found in *Values Clarification* (Simon et al., 1972). The log serves as a structure for the discussion during the supervision session although the log per se may be kept in confidence by the supervisee.

Supervisors using the various self-report techniques assume that the supervisee has the ability to identify and label thoughts and feelings and to verbalize them with the supervisor. Some supervisees may need other techniques to help them increase their insight and affective sensitivity.

Role-playing

Role-playing is a technique that stimulates supervisee thoughts and feelings in a relatively safe environment; the thoughts and feelings are then examined by the supervisor and supervisees as they relate to those experienced by the supervisee in interpersonal relationships. Two basic formats exist for role-playing in the Personal Growth model of supervision. One format is for the supervisee to play the role of a person who displays a particular attitude, personality characteristic, or behavior that is unfamiliar to or uncomfortable for the supervisee. The objective is to have the supervisee understand the feelings and thoughts of a certain type of person by role-playing that person. For example, a supervisee may have had little experience with very lonely persons, so the supervisee would role-play a lonely person in order to increase insight in and affective sensitivity to lonely people. The supervisor's role is to maintain a personal but nonprofessional conversation with the supervisee allowing the direction of the conversation to be controlled by the supervisee. Following the brief role-play, the supervisor and supervisee discuss the role-play focusing on the ideas and emotions experienced by the supervisee.

The second format for role-playing in the Personal Growth model of supervision is for the supervisor to role-play a person with a certain attitude or behavior and have the supervisee follow along in a nonprofessional/nontherapeutic conversation. The purpose of this role-play format is to have the supervisee become aware of ideas and feelings toward an unfamiliar or uncomfortable type of person by interacting with that person. For example, the supervisee may be unaware of the hostility in some persons. The supervisor would role-play such a person in order to have the supervisee experience thoughts and feelings that are then discussed after the role-play.

In both role-play formats the participants assume they are in a nonprofessional encounter and so may portray co-workers, neighbors, acquaintances at a social gathering or any context other than a professional/clinical setting. Role-playing a nonprofessional situation in the Personal Growth model reduces the pressure on the supervisee to produce the professionally-appropriate idea or feeling. In the Skill Development model the reactions of the supervisee role-playing a clinician are critiqued after the role-play, thereby adding an evaluative dimension that does not occur during the role-playing in the Personal Growth model.

The supervisor does have impressions and emotional reactions to the supervisee during the role-play and may share these ideas and feelings he or she experienced during the role-play directly with the supervisee. In this feedback process the supervisor attempts to provide data to the supervisee that can be assimilated and used for increased insight and affective sensitivity. Although the supervisor models some degree of insight and sensitivity by providing feedback, which is helpful, the intrinsically evaluative nature of the supervisor's feedback can threaten the supervisee.

Supervisees who need additional structure can be directed to books such as *Values Clarification* (Simon et al., 1972) or *Personalizing Education* (Howe & Howe, 1975). The topics in these books consist of personal questions such as "To what extent do I spend my leisure time with others or by myself?" or incomplete sentences such as "If I were angry at my boss, I would. . . ."

Supervisees might also be directed to describe feelings that are found in one or more of the categories and subcategories listed and described by Hackney and Cormier (1979) in *Counseling Strategies and Objectives*. For example, the category of affection includes enjoyment, competence, love, happiness, and hope. Supervisees may also be trained to discriminate among feelings and between thoughts and feelings by completing the exercises found in Egan's *Exercises in Helping Skills* (1975) and in Hackney and Cormier's (1979) text.

The role-playing usually produces a wealth of ideas and feelings within the supervisee that can be compared to ideas and feelings experienced with other people. With the focus on relationships outside the professional setting, the supervisee begins to identify patterns of relationships that had not been previously identified or to identify the feelings experienced in various interpersonal situations.

Group Work

Abels (1977) characterized all types of supervisory groups by stating, "Group supervision can offer an opportunity for a supportive community whose norms of mutual aid and client service permit only the best in practice to develop" (p. 198). The personal growth group, in particular, is a frequently used technique in which supervisees meet on a regular basis to discuss their ideas and feelings about themselves. Unlike the group discussion and the case conference used in the Skill Development model, the personal growth group is focused on ideas and feelings of supervisees about themselves and their relationships with people outside their immediate professional roles. The group goal is to increase insight and affective sensitivity rather than improve clinical techniques or approaches as in the case conference and group discussion.

Advantages of group work for supervisees include emotional support, "normalization" of ideas and feelings, and awareness of different points of view about effective interpersonal relations. Although emotional support for a supervisee is certainly found in individual supervision, for some supervisees the support of peers is especially powerful. Also, the support of several persons may be more helpful than the support of a single supervisor. Closely related to emotional support is "normalization," that is, when supervisees realize that they are not alone or unusual in their ideas and feelings as supervisees share experiences. Of course, not all of the supervisees' experiences are identical and so supervisees gain a variety of suggestions and examples of interpersonal behavior. The group generates support and provides new ideas for supervisees to consider.

Students often participate in personal growth groups during their university training to become aware of the role of a group member and the feelings accompanied by such membership. This understanding and emotional sensitivity helps students to understand more clearly the thoughts and feelings of participants in groups that students eventually will lead.

Disadvantages of group work in supervision are similar to disadvantages in any type of clinical group work: a low level of trust may be present; the group may wander from the task; participants may fear negative evaluations by the leader. All of these situations can decrease the effectiveness of group work.

Several steps can reduce or eliminate the pitfalls mentioned above, and those steps are described by Gazda (1971), Lakin (1972), Yalom (1975), and Ohlsen (1977). To increase trust, the group can meet on a frequent and regularly-scheduled basis. Also, specific exercises can be conducted to increase participants' self-disclosures in order to encourage acceptance and trust of each other. Activities can be found in many books such as the volumes of *A Handbook of Structured Experiences for Human Relations Training* by Pfeiffer and Jones (1969). Personal growth groups will be improved by the establishment of specific goals and the use of a structured format to accomplish those goals. Research by Cormier et al. (1974), Levin and Kurtz (1974), and Gormally (1975) confirm that personal growth groups can be improved through increased structure.

When supervisees are led in a growth group by the person who is also their individual supervisor, many supervisees fear a negative evaluation by the supervisor if they reveal ideas or feelings that seem inappropriate. Of course, it may be helpful for the supervisees to "work through" this fear; however, the situation could be avoided thus allowing more time for other topics by having the group led by a faculty or staff member other than the individual supervisor.

Research in psychology has shown that personal growth groups have produced changes among students-in-training in terms of self-understanding (McKinnon, 1969), self-recognition (Apostal & Muro, 1970), and improved interpersonal relationships among each other (Banikotes, 1975). Personal growth groups will likely continue as a primary technique of accomplishing the goals of the Personal Growth model of supervision.

Peers

Clinicians in training or on the job can effectively supervise each other, either in pairs (Wagner & Smith, 1979) or in peer groups (Todd & Pine, 1968; Allen, 1976) without a designated supervisor. As described in more detail in Chapter 3, the rationale for using peer supervision is that peers will offer support, make suggestions, and self-disclose more freely without a supervisor present because they will have fewer feelings of apprehension about the supervisor's negative evaluation of them. As in the Skill Development and Integration models of supervision, peer group supervision in the Personal Growth model depends on the peers' perception of themselves as relatively similar in skills and personal development. Although some question this similarity and the actual reduction of evaluation apprehension via peer supervision, the technique has some definite potential as an effective supervisory technique.

The effectiveness of peer supervision will be determined, in part, by the ability of the peers to adhere to the goals established and their ability to alternate between the roles of supervisor and supervisee throughout the supervision process. The faculty or staff member who organizes the peer supervision should carefully instruct the peer dyads about the goals of insight and affective sensitivity and the inappropriateness of turning supervision into therapy. Furthermore, the faculty or staff member should train the supervisees in the roles of supervisor and supervisee that each will need to adopt as Wagner and Smith (1979) did with their supervisees. Then, as the peers begin to work with each other, the faculty or staff member should meet with the dyads on a periodic basis, even examining a tape of a peer supervision session, to ensure that the appropriate goals are being worked on, that suitable progress is being attained, and that each person is taking the role of supervisor and supervisee as the process continues.

The monitoring of the peers by a person outside the supervisory dyad, such as a faculty or staff member, may arouse some feelings of fear or resentment among the peers that is counterproductive to their growth. If the peers do not follow the goals that are established, however, of if one peer initially assumes and maintains the supervisor role in the dyad, the peer supervision process will be ineffective. Wagner and Smith (1979) monitored the peer dyads very closely and reported large gains by this technique, thus suggesting that any feelings of resistance by the peers toward the supervisors were not detrimental to any noticeable degree.

In groups of peers, as in dyads, the supervisees need careful instruction in the goals of insight and affective sensitivity and in the roles of supervisor and supervisee. Generally, the principles of leaderless groups apply (Yalom, 1975) where some peers assume a supervisor/helper role and others take on a supervisee/helpee position. Groups that are effective must be flexible regarding roles so that all members can, at various times, experience the supervisee role. Groups must also maintain an effective balance between roles within each group session because everyone cannot be a supervisor (or a supervisee) at any one point in time. If too many people take supervisee roles, little support or new ideas will be provided. As with peer dyads, periodic evaluation by a faculty or staff member outside the peer group could correct any difficulties.

Peer supervision is a potentially useful supervisory technique that has not, as yet, been examined carefully for its effects on supervisee development. Research to assess peer supervision in the Personal Growth model must rely on the areas of human relations development and group work as well as supervision in order to help supervisors know how and for whom this new technique can best be applied.

Observation

In the Personal Growth model the supervisory technique of observation (as well as sitting-in and review of tape recordings) allows the supervisor to view directly the reactions of the supervisee to persons other than the supervisor. In this way the supervisor gains valuable data that confirm or disconfirm ideas about the supervisee because the supervisee may act in some ways that are similar and some ways that are dissimilar to the behavior displayed during supervision. The supervisor can use this information indirectly by focusing the supervisee's attention to areas suggested by the observations made by the supervisor. In this way the observation session has helped the supervisor to understand the supervisee better, which helps the supervisor to assist the supervisee in gaining insight and affective sensitivity. A more direct use of the data gained by the supervisor through the observation technique is for the supervisor to share selected impressions and reactions of the supervisee with the supervisee in the supervision session. For feedback of this type to be effective, a clear understanding must be established between supervisor and supervisee about what types of information the supervisor will share with the supervisee and how this information will be used to promote personal growth.

Observation can be improved by using rating scales or other structured assessment forms that are related to the issues that the supervisor and supervisee have agreed to examine. For example, the supervisor may have agreed to observe the supervisee's behavior to note any signs of over protectiveness. The supervisor could write down any phrases the supervisee used toward the client indicating this tendency. Following the observed session, the supervisor could meet with the supervisee in a supervision session. The supervisor might guide the supervisee in a Socratic manner into an introspective exploration of the overprotection issue as it is manifested in interpersonal relations, or the supervisor may give specific observations of the supervisee's behavior, which suggests an over protective position, quickly followed by a broader discussion of when, how, and with whom the supervisee may be overprotective. The goals of the supervisor are the same in both instances but the data are used in different ways.

When feedback is given by a supervisor to a supervisee about a session the supervisor has observed through a one-way mirror (or another method), the feedback should be given as soon after the therapy session as possible. Research by Doyle, Foreman, and Wales (1977) compared feedback given in immediate supervision and delayed supervision and found that learning was greater when provided immediately after the supervisee's observed session with a client. When the supervisor does not give specific feedback and uses the data gained from an observed therapy session in a more indirect way, however, the supervision session does not have to follow the therapy session immediately. Delayed supervision might be more effective than immediate supervision if the supervisee used the time between the therapy session and the supervision session to reflect on specific behaviors, attitudes, and feelings aroused during the therapy session. Quite clearly the effective use of observation must be considered in light of the approach of the supervisor in increasing the insight and affective sensitivity of the supervisee.

Sitting-in

Sitting-in is a technique, as described in Chapter 3, in which the supervisor sits in a therapy session conducted by the supervisee. This technique is used typically with beginning supervisees in training programs during some of their initial interviews. Used in this way the technique may provide emotional support for a novice clinician, could allow the supervisor to model effective clinical behavior, and may gain valuable data for the supervisor to use in the supervision session conducted later.

In the Personal Growth model, sitting-in is used to provide the supervisor with information about the behavior of the supervisee that can be used later in supervision to increase the supervisee's insight and/or affective sensitivity. Consequently, sitting-in is used usually as a substitute for observation when a room with a one-way mirror is not available. Because considerably more anxiety is apt to be aroused by sitting-in than by observation (or tape review), the supervisee's behavior will be atypical.

Sitting-in should be used within the Personal Growth model only when the supervisor and supervisee plan the topics the supervisor will observe and how the data gained will be used in supervision. Furthermore, the supervisor should remain silent while sitting-in because the purpose of the technique in the Personal Growth model is to gain information and provide support, not to model techniques, or correct the technique of the supervisee. Sitting-in may also be used at points other than with a supervisee's initial sessions, but the purpose remains the same.

Once the supervisee has gained some confidence in clinical skills, the supervisor can plan to sit-in on a variety of clients who are at various points in their therapy with the supervisee. Sitting in on sessions other than initial ones allows the supervisor to see the supervisee in interpersonal relations that call for and permit different behavior than that displayed in initial interviews. All of these procedures for the use of the sitting-in technique will allow the supervisor to stay within the Personal Growth model of supervision.

Audiotape and Videotape Recordings

Although commonly applied in the Skill Development model, tape recordings can be used to help supervisees gain insight and affective sensitivity through the Personal Growth model. In contrast to using tape review for building skills or case conceptualizations, as in the Skill Development model, using the Personal Growth model helps the supervisee to move into an exploration of interpersonal relationships with persons other than clients. Tape recordings, at a simple level, can be reviewed by the supervisor for information about the supervisee's behavior outside of supervision. This information can be helpful in directing the supervisor's efforts toward particular ideas and feelings of the supervisee. Furthermore, the supervisor can select and, during the supervision, play segments of a tape that will stimulate discussion of the supervisee's behavior. Not only does a supervisor have examples of the supervisee's behavior, which is also true of the observation and sitting-in techniques, but also the supervisor can replay these examples exactly as they occurred. Tape review is particularly effective because the supervisee is away from the therapy session and can reflect on the example without pressure to make an appropriate clinical response to a client.

As in the Skill Development and Integration models, greater benefit will be achieved with tape review if both supervisee and supervisor review the tape before the supervision session so they can thoughtfully prepare themselves. Supervisees should consider how thoughts and feelings toward the client are similar to and different from their reactions to other persons in their lives. Supervisors should look for reactions of the supervisees to the client that suggest thoughts that are unclear or feelings that are inappropriate, extreme, or perhaps missing. The supervisor then focuses on the supervisee's views of relationships and feelings with others as suggested by the situations on the tape. Anderson and Brown (1955) give an excellent anecdotal description of tape review as a technique for enhancing personal growth.

Co-therapy

Co-therapy is another means of increasing supervisees' personal growth and is applied by means of one of two basic formats. In one format a supervisee is paired with an individual supervisor as a co-therapist to learn how to work with a group or family. The discussion following each therapy session conducted by these co-therapists, however, can be focused by the supervisor on the personal growth of the supervisee. The supervisor helps the supervisee identify and clarify the supervisee's behavior patterns and feelings that were prompted by the therapy session. Like sitting-in, this type of co-therapy allows for the supervisor to have first-hand information about the supervisee. Furthermore, the supervisor and supervisee can develop more mutual respect and trust as colleagues by working together than they would by sitting-in, observation, or tape review. Working together allows supervisor and supervisee the opportunity to take on different roles (colleagues) from those typically assumed by supervisors and supervisees, thus permitting increased respect for each other's clinical competence and trust in each other's personal behavior. This increased respect and trust allows the supervisor to move into sensitive issues more quickly than he or she would be able to using other techniques or other formats for co-therapy.

Another format for co-therapy supervision is having two clinicians (either students or regular staff members) work together as co-therapists while being supervised by a third person, usually their individual supervisor (Tucker et al., 1976). The co-therapists conduct a therapy session that the supervisor may observe directly or review by means of a tape made by the co-therapists. The supervisor then meets with both co-therapists in a supervision session. (An alternative procedure would be for the supervisor to meet with each co-therapist individually or to blend the individual and joint meetings.) Another variation is to use the peer supervision idea and have the co-therapists meet with each other and later meet as a group with their supervisor.

The intense nature of co-therapist relations stimulates many behavior patterns and feelings that can be explored with the supervisor. The supervisor compares the relationship between the co-therapists with their actions and feelings in other relationships. As shown by the powerful results of those using co-therapy in working with couples and groups, co-therapy in supervision has exciting possibilities for developing the personal growth of the supervisee.

APPLICATION OF THE PERSONAL GROWTH MODEL

The Personal Growth model is widely applicable to students and clinicians in the field and is designed to increase their insight and affective sensitivity about interpersonal relationships. The primary assumption of this model is that a supervisee who becomes, in general, more insightful and sensitive will also become more effective with clients. The techniques used to accomplish the goals of the Personal Growth model are similar in form to those used in other models, but the application varies greatly from model to model. Several guidelines are given here to help supervisors apply the Personal Growth model followed by an evaluation of the model that includes key issues facing the model.

Guidelines

The first guideline is to thoroughly discuss the differences between personal growth activities in supervision for educative purposes and therapy with the supervisee. Once the supervisee clearly understands that the emphasis of the Personal Growth model is enhancement of existing levels of growth, not remediation or conflict-resolution as in therapy, the supervisee may feel more comfortable with the supervisor's role and techniques. More specifically, the supervisee may feel less evaluation apprehension toward the supervisor and thus respond with increased honesty and openness. The supervisee should realize that the supervisor will not probe the defenses of the supervisee and will not look for hidden problems. Also, the supervisor will prevent the supervisee from initiating such a therapeutic process. This agreement allows the supervisee freedom to be introspective without fear of getting "too deep," that is, learning information that is anxiety-provoking or losing emotional control—all fears of people engaged in self-exploration. Personal change can occur without a therapist, however. A supervisee may act on insights gained in supervision, for example, by changing certain interpersonal behavior with others, but there is no requirement to do so, as in therapy, in order to resolve a conflict or remedy a deficiency.

Another guideline is to discuss the goals of the Personal Growth model—increasing insight and affective sensitivity—with the supervisee. Some supervisors emphasize insight and others emphasize affective sensitivity; therefore, the supervisor should describe any such emphasis to the supervisee. Furthermore, the use and definition of either goal allows the supervisee to conceptualize personal growth in more concrete terms. The clearer the supervisee understands either goal of the Personal Growth model, the more likely it is that the goal will be attained.

An additional guideline is to describe the techniques that will be used (or are likely to be used) throughout the supervisory process in order to prepare the supervisee for future sessions. In this way the supervisee knows the technique and the purpose for using it before the technique is implemented. This guideline allows the supervisor to reduce the supervisee's fears of the unknown and eliminate surprises—always anxiety-provoking to a supervisee. Of course, some anxiety is inevitable but high anxiety can and should be avoided by the guidelines listed here.

Another guideline to remember is that techniques can be helpful in gathering data, but the data must be processed between supervisor and supervisee in order to enhance personal growth. The processing or discussion between supervisor and supervisee is the most important aspect of any supervisory technique used in the Personal Growth model. In this regard supervisors should consider the point at which the supervisory discussion session should follow a therapy session or sessions conducted by the supervisee. When the supervision session immediately follows a therapy session, the supervisee is most keenly aware of thoughts and feelings that occurred during the session. Supervisees, however, are sometimes too stimulated by feelings aroused during the therapy session to reflect on their general interpersonal functioning. Also, supervisees often want to focus on skills and client conceptualization when the supervision session immediately follows a therapy session. For these persons delayed supervision is advisable. In delayed supervision, the supervisor meets with the supervisee a few hours or a few days after a clinical session has been conducted. In this way the supervisee will have had time to reflect on insights and feelings about in-session behavior and general interpersonal behavior.

One final guideline is to begin the personal growth process in supervision through structured activities that give discrete information to supervisees about specific interpersonal behavior. The idea is to use aids such as checklists or journals to gather data that is directly related to the goals that have been established. Research studies have clearly shown the wishes of supervisees for structure during the beginning of supervision, thus suggesting a value in structuring the personal growth activities that are conducted.

Evaluation

The Personal Growth model of supervision has not been clearly assessed apart from the emotional support and growth that occur within all models of supervision (Nash, 1975). The Personal Growth model as described in this chapter, however, is designed to go beyond the incidental emotional support and growth that occur in a random manner. Survey research by Doehrman (1976) and anecdotal reports of supervisees (Nelson, 1978) suggest that the Personal Growth model is very powerful. Empirical research summarized by Hansen and Warner (1971) and Hansen, et al. (1976) shows little examination of the Personal Growth model. Once field researchers have more carefully delineated the effects of the Personal Growth model, such as increased open-mindedness (Mezzano, 1969), empirical research can be done to measure these effects on clinician-client interactions and client change.

Doehrman (1976) provides the strongest support for the Personal Growth model through her extensive study of the reciprocal effects of supervision and psychotherapy among advanced doctoral students during their internship. In this landmark study Doehrman traced the impasses in supervision to specific conflicts that occurred in supervisees' therapy sessions. Conversely, she showed how impasses between supervisees and clients were related to interactions that had occurred in supervision sessions. The supervisors used the Personal Growth model in their work, which Doehrman measured in terms of the feelings and insights the supervisees gained toward clients and toward their supervisors. Like most studies of the Personal Growth model, Doehrman's examines the self-reports of supervisors and supervisees (a usually biased source of data). She then made inferences about the phenomena occurring between supervisor and supervisee and their relationship to the phenomena occurring between supervisee and client.

Although data-gathering via means such as a rating scale and a structured interview are quite acceptable to researchers with a phenomenological theory of human behavior, the form does not meet the rigors of the procedures used by behaviorists or researchers with a behavioral theory. Furthermore, Doehrman made inferences about the relationship between what happens in supervision (e.g.. roles taken, issues discussed, feelings toward each other) and subsequent events in therapy. Although there can be no definitive cause and effect relationship established in an empirical sense, Doehrman presents evidence that is difficult to dismiss. Consistently, the activities between supervisor and supervisee seem to affect the behavior of the supervisee in therapy sessions with clients. Conversely, the activities in therapy seem to affect the supervisee's behavior in supervision sessions. Such data cannot be dismissed as post-hoc speculation, and it needs to be examined with the rigor used in other psychological studies.

As studies of the Personal Growth model become more structured, several tasks must be accomplished. One task is to increase the size of the sample so that statements can be made with confidence about the general effects of the model. When studies are conducted on a few supervisors and supervisees, there is the danger that the results, whether positive or negative, are idiosyncratic and so cannot be generalized to other groups. Furthermore, researchers examining the Personal Growth model must be willing to add measurement strategies that rely on observable behavior to the self-report strategies currently in use. This task is not designed to bridge the theoretical gap between behaviorists and phenomenologists but to increase the confidence about which inferences can be made regarding the model. It is hoped that researchers of all theoretical persuasions can examine the Personal Growth model and establish a clearer understanding of its effects.

A criticism of the Personal Growth model, as well as of the Skill Development model, is that it may encourage dependence on the supervisor. The important issue is whether supervisors, regardless of the model, allow or encourage supervisees to become dependent on them either for emotional support via the Personal Growth model or for direction as in the Skill Development model. Supervisors encourage dependence by directly or indirectly communicating that supervisees are not yet competent in terms of skills or interpersonal functioning to make independent decisions. Consequently, supervisees who accept this message may become dependent on the supervisor. This message to supervisees is facilitated by a supervisor who emphasizes the role of the supervisee as novice and that of the supervisor as expert—the hierarchy between them. Supervisors who emphasize, directly or indirectly, their greater level of skill or personal development may increase dependency with some supervisees but may create counter dependency in others. In the latter case certain supervisees may react quite negatively to the supervisor's emphasis on the hierarchy between them and may become resistant to further learning in supervision. If dependency can be a problem, as is frequently described, counterdependency would seem to be an equally likely problem.

A criticism more particular to the Personal Growth model is that it is used by supervisors who don't know what else to do with supervisees. Supervisors may be comfortable and adept at providing emotional support and directing a supervisee in personal growth activities because these activities are close to the therapy approach in which the supervisors have been trained. Without training as supervisors, they may lack the knowledge and skills of achieving skill development or integration. Consequently, they implement the Personal Growth model as the only option open to them.

A subtle aspect of the Personal Growth model and the Skill Development model is that there is always more that can be done. If personal growth (or skills or integration) is placed on a continuum with no endpoint, then one's level of development could always increase and so supervisors would be justified in continuing to use the Personal Growth (or Skill Development or Integration) model indefinitely. Research on the developmental process of supervision suggests, however, that supervisees want skills, personal growth, and integration, not just one model. Using only one model throughout supervision may be more for the comfort of the supervisor than for the benefit of the supervisee.

Perhaps the biggest criticism is that the Personal Growth model is not directly tied to observable behavior change by the supervisee with clients. Although this criticism is not based on research evidence, it continues to be expressed. A more appropriate criticism is that advocates of this model have not, as yet, examined (except for Doehrman, 1976) the results of the model on supervisees' interactions with clients. One suggestion is that researchers look for effects rather than seek to prove whether certain effects, chosen on an a priori basis, are present. It is assumed in this text that significant interactions will occur between supervisor and supervisee in all models of supervision and that these interactions will have effects on supervisees' behavior with other people, some of whom are clients.

Supervisors can, and some do, adopt an extreme or purist view and say that to accept the personal growth view is unjustified by facts and that only supervisory interactions proved effective in causing client change are important. The retort is that the science of human behavior is imprecise and many interactions occur that cannot, as yet, be measured for their effects on the overt behavior of others. It is equally inappropriate to have a single criterion for supervisee success whether the criterion is increased supervisee personal growth or acquisition of therapeutic skills and knowledge, and so supervisors should consider using both criteria.

The Personal Growth model is used frequently with more advanced supervisees who have achieved some moderate level of skill development and wish (or are urged by their supervisor) to increase their insight or emotional sensitivity. These supervisees have gained some confidence in their ability as clinicians and can allow themselves to examine their own interpersonal behavior and responses with the ultimate goal of being able to use their previously learned skills and knowledge in a more effective manner. The Personal Growth model is a powerful form of supervision and, although its effects are not yet clearly specified, it is applicable in a wide variety of settings.

SUMMARY

The Personal Growth model is based on the assumption that supervisees who develop a high degree of effective interpersonal functioning will be better able to use the skills that have been previously taught in formal courses, workshops, readings, and other means and will be more effective in relationships with clients. Although this assumption is consistent with tenets of a phenomenological orientation to therapy, supervisors of any theoretical orientation toward clinical practice may adopt the assumption that supervisees need effective interpersonal behavior in order to use specific clinical skills with success.

The Personal Growth model is designed to achieve the goals of increased insight and/or increased affective sensitivity of the supervisee. These goals are achieved by collecting data about the supervisee's behavior through various supervisory techniques and discussing the behavior patterns and emotional reactions of the supervisee in interpersonal relationships that occur outside the professional/clinical realm. The Personal Growth model is usually applied with more advanced supervisees and is probably used when few constraints exist on the length of time supervision will last. Although little experimental research has been conducted on this model, survey research and anecdotal reports suggest this model is valuable and powerful. In the future, researchers must specify the effects of supervision as differentiated from the effects of the personal relationship between supervisor and supervisee and must measure the effects of the model in terms of the behavior change of the supervisee with clients.

Chapter 5

Integration Model

DESCRIPTION OF THE MODEL

A third model of supervision—the Integration model—is one frequently used by supervisors of advanced students or experienced agency clinicians. It provides a goal for supervision that is different from, but clearly complimentary to, the goals of the Skill Development and Personal Growth models. As the name suggests, this model builds on the previous knowledge of the supervisee and so has the potential for assisting supervisees to become maximally effective in their clinical activities.

The goal of the Integration model is to integrate the supervisee's present skills and case conceptualization with existing levels of sensitivity and insight. In this way all the resources of a supervisee are brought together to a particular case so that the developing clinician understands the effects of knowledge, therapeutic skills, and personal attributes on his or her clients. Often, beginning clinicians (and many experienced clinicians also) believe that client change is based on one or two particular skills or personal attributes and they tend to overlook the Gestalt of their interaction with clients. To attribute client change to only a few characteristics oversimplifies human interactions. Perhaps clinicians (and researchers) who believe in the power of a single traumatic incident in a client's life also believe in the power of a particular skill or attribute in therapy. The supervisor who utilizes the Integration model believes that the skills and personal growth of a therapist must be integrated so that their combined impact—not one or the other—is brought to bear on clients.

The process carried out in the Integration model is best described as "collaborative." Collaborative implies a mutual endeavor between persons whose functional relationship is like that of peers. In supervision the supervisor and supervisee meet as different-but-equal professionals who mutually examine issues in order to integrate the previously learned therapeutic skills with the previously acquired personal development in order to help a particular client. This description may seem similar to the process of consultation; but, as described in Chapter 1, consultation and supervision differ significantly. A consultant is presumed to have particular knowledge or expertise not possessed by the consultee, and the consultee is presumed to be operating in his or her own sphere independent of the consultant, free to accept or reject the consultant's advice, and under no obligation to implement suggestions or to report back on their effects. Even though the model of supervision described in this chapter has been referred to as a "consultation" model (Hart

131

et al., 1976a, 1976b, 1976c; Kurpius & Baker, 1977; Gurk & Wicas, 1979), the term *collaborative* seems to fit more precisely.

Like the Skill Development and Personal Growth models, the Integration model differs from other models according to 1) the functional relationship of the participants, 2) their hierarchical distance, and 3) the focus of the supervision sessions. In the Integration model the supervisor's functional relationship is that of a knowledgeable and skilled colleague whose primary importance lies in contributing a different (not necessarily better) point of view from that of the supervisee. The supervisor's job is not to add skills or personal development to the supervisee but to bring the supervisee's existing skills and sensitivity to bear on particular clients with whom the supervisee is presently working. The supervisee has expertise and the desire to use this expertise in an effective manner with a particular client. Together, supervisor and supervisee share information, form hypotheses, and evaluate the behavior of the supervisee and the client.

Sources of power in interpersonal relations, originally described by French and Raven (1960), were applied to supervision by Kadushin (1976). Supervisors who adopt the collegial or collaborator role rely primarily on the relationship between them (referent power) to motivate the supervisee to share in the examination of clinical sessions, the finding of solutions, and the evaluation of the supervisee's professional behavior. Referent power is illustrated by the belief of the supervisor and supervisee that "We are in the same profession, sharing similar aims and concerns, so let's work together." Supervisors using the Skill Development model, in contrast to those using the Integration model, adopt the role of teacher, and in the Personal Growth model, they accept a therapist role. In both of these roles supervisors rely mostly on the power of their clinical expertise (expert power) or their administrative position (positional power) in order to influence supervisee skills or insight and affective sensitivity

In many ways the supervisor and supervisee using the Integration model have a peer relationship. The supervisor, however, usually has some evaluative function regarding the supervisee's progress in the training program or in the agency, and this function prevents supervisors and supervisees from ever attaining a true peer or colleague relationship. Yet, the somewhat egalitarian relationship of the Integration model is designed to reduce supervisee fear of being criticized for failing to meet the standards of an omnipotent supervisor or of shame for disappointing an admired supervisor. When supervisor and supervisee work as team members rather than as leader and member, the supervisee feels independent of the supervisor and thus more confident about the interactions with the supervisor. As Nash (1975) concluded from her research, "Supervisors who are perceived as exercising authority in a collaborative way are preferred [by supervisees]; with them students feel able to learn and grow" (p. 106).

Furthermore, the collaborative relationship is designed to help the supervisee develop an internal sense of evaluation to replace the external sense of evaluation previously acquired through the critera for acceptable performance established by university or agency and transmitted by the supervisor. Criteria may reflect specific skills, conceptual knowledge, personal attributes, or ethical standards ranging from specific behavioral standards to vague principles. Unless the criteria are internalized, however, it is unlikely that supervisees will continue to meet them after supervision is concluded. Through a collaborative relationship the supervisee is encouraged, with the aid of the supervisor, to develop personal criteria for professional competence.

The second dimension that differentiates models of supervision is the hierarchical distance between supervisor and supervisee. The hierarchical distance in the Integration model is generally low and is less than the distance in the Skill Development and Personal Growth models. A reduced hierarchy between supervisor and supervisee encourages the supervisee to become more active and responsible during supervision. Furthermore, supervisees often feel less pressure from the supervisor to perform without errors, which encourages self-confidence about working with new and difficult cases. Supervisees will realize that such cases will allow them to learn and even though errors occur, learning will take place.

The third dimension that differentiates the Integration model from other models of supervision is the focus of the session. In the Integration model the supervisor and supervisee focus on the supervisee's interpersonal relationship with clients. Typically, the supervisor examines the supervisee's behavior, attitudes, and feelings toward a specific individual client, family, or group. In contrast to the Skill Development model in which the supervisor focuses on the supervisee's conceptualization of and specific supervisee interventions with a client, in the Integration model, the supervisor examines the result of those conceptualizations and interventions in terms of patterns in which the supervisee and client are engaged. These patterns are able to be differentiated in terms of their impact on the effectiveness of the therapeutic process.

An important aspect of the focus in the Integration model is the unit that is examined. The supervisee and the client are viewed as a mutually interdependent unit in which each affects the other.

This dyadic unit is seen as an ongoing cyclical interaction not as a linear action-reaction of only the supervisee's intervention to the client as is typically the view when using the Skill Development and Personal Growth models.

Although the systemic or ecological viewpoint could be adopted by a supervisor whose goal is to increase skill development, virtually all supervisors take a more one-dimensional focus. That is, supervisors using the Skill Development model typically help supervisees to see the results of their interactions in terms of client response—a linear, cause and effect system. A similar situation exists for supervisors using the Personal Growth model in that they typically assist supervisees to develop sensitivity and insight without considering the impact of the client on the supervisee. Although supervisors with a systemic framework might use either the Skill Development or Personal Growth models, the goal of the Integration model may be more inherently consistent with the systemic view and so attracts supervisors with this framework.

This focus in the Integration model has been called a process focus by Ekstein and Wallerstein (1958) who described a way of approaching the supervisee-client interaction in a therapist-like fashion. Abroms supported this viewpoint by calling it metatherapy. He stated, "supervision is a relationship between a supervisor and a therapeutic relationship. Its aim is metatherapeutic: to promote changes in the therapist-client relationship" (Abroms, 1977, p. 83). This focus clearly differentiates the Integration model from other models of supervision.

One other aspect that is part of the focus by supervisors using the Integration model is the powerful effect that clients, supervisees, and supervisors have on each other, which was first described by Searles (1955) as the reflection process. "The processes at work currently in the relationship between patient and therapist are often reflected in the relationship between therapist and supervisor," Searles (1955, p. 135) said. Doehrman's (1976) study documents this phenomenon and, in addition, how the relationship between supervisor and supervisee is reflected in the relationship between supervisee and client. Doehrman used the term *parallel process*. Mueller and Kell (1972) described in greater detail how the anxiety from the supervisor, supervisee, or client causes impasses to develop between supervisor and supervisee or between supervisee and client. Particular importance is placed on the impasse that develops initially between supervisee and client and how this impasse can be resolved in supervision.

Indeed, resolution of impasses becomes the central focus of supervision for Mueller and Kell (1972).

According to our paradigm of supervision, all three sources of conflict and anxiety—the client in relation to others, the client and therapist in relation to each other, and the therapist and supervisor in relation to each other—must find their way into the supervisory relationship if it is to be productive. The way in which the supervisor interacts with the therapist or assists him to cope with the conflict generated in each of these relationships as the conflicts unfold, merge, and interact, defines the supervisory process. Unless all three sources of conflict and their interaction become a part of the process, supervision will provide no new dimensions to the development of the therapist that can't be obtained with less expenditure of time, energy, and emotional commitment elsewhere (Mueller & Kell, 1972, p. 7).

In the Integration model supervisors who use the parallel process concept will greatly strengthen supervisees' understanding of interactional patterns and help supervisees to resolve their impasses with clients. Other similar reports by supervisors would be helpful to colleagues needing specific suggestions. Videotapes by Hart (1974, 1976d, 1976e) show supervisees describing their impasses.

Authors from psychiatry, including Rosenbaum (1953) and Ekstein and Wallerstein (1958), studied the "process oriented" focus and found this focus to be clearly different from a focus on the patient or on the growth of the clinician. This focus is not the *what* of the clinician's work (techniques, approaches) nor the *who* of the clinician (personality, attitudes, feelings, general interpersonal behavior), but it is the *how* of the clinician's professional interactions. Each clinician acts in characteristic ways with clients that are somewhat different from interpersonal patterns with people in general. These characteristic behaviors evolve from an integration of theories of therapy and human behavior, experience as a professional, role expectations conveyed by the university, the agency, and society, and the clinician's general interpersonal patterns. The knowledge acquired in training programs about therapy and human behavior is tested in clinical experiences, and along with feedback from these experiences help to form a clinician's patterns. These patterns are also shaped by the clinician's expectation of how to behave as communicated by faculty members, colleagues, professional organizations, and recipients of the services. The combined impact of these influences produces a person who behaves differently from the person not undergoing this educational process. The overall intent of the Integration model is to help the supervisee to become aware of and effectively apply the characteristic patterns of therapeutic knowledge/techniques and personal behavior.

An assumption of the Integration model is that supervisees have mastery of therapeutic skills and some minimal level of personal growth but do not display a consistent or integrated application of these two components to professional interactions. A thorough review of the supervision literature led Kurpius and Baker (1977) to support the idea that the Integration model is used with students who have attained some level of skill and personal growth. "There is a suggestion in the literature that consultation [Integration model] becomes a more dominant mode of supervision as the trainee becomes increasingly able and professional in his performance" (Kurpius & Baker, 1977, p. 228). The level of skills a supervisee is expected to possess depends on the level of the student's training (paraprofessional to post-doctoral) and the professional duties assigned to the clinician. Supervisors will not expect as much from supervisees who are less well-trained and who conduct less complex and demanding duties as they will from supervisees who are more highly trained or who work in more difficult professional situations. Similarly, supervisors expect some minimal level of personal growth as suggested by a supervisee's experiences in training and in life. A 21-year-old, beginning mental health worker will not be expected to have the insight and affective sensitivity of an older person who has had more opportunities for personal growth via formal and informal means. Of course, no supervisor can rely on a linear relationship between supervisee age, experience, or years of training and level of supervisee skill or personal growth and should be prepared for exceptions to this formula.

Regardless of the supervisee's level of skills or personal growth, the supervisor using the Integration model focuses on professional situations for which the supervisee possesses the necessary skills and personal growth. If the supervisee seems to need additional skills or insight and affective sensitivity of a general nature, the supervisor may change to a different model of supervision or refer the supervisee to another source for additional assistance. If the supervisee has the appropriate level of skills and personal development for the assigned duties and client population, the supervisor using the Integration model will focus on the application of the supervisee's skills, rather than add new skills or increase the supervisee's personal growth. This sequence of supervisory tasks from skill acquisition to application is parallel to the sequence of therapeutic skills advocated by Cleghorn and Levin (1973) in which basic objectives are differentiated from advanced objectives. The Integration model consists of advanced objectives that rely on the attainment of the basic objectives of skill development and personal growth.

Furthermore, the supervisor implementing the Integration model helps supervisees integrate their techniques into their interpersonal relationship style. The goal is for supervisees to use techniques as a natural and authentic part of their interpersonal relationships. Many beginning supervisees use techniques in an awkward and mechanistic way that makes clients feel like objects that are being manipulated. In order to achieve integration, supervisors and supervisees must first identify the approaches and techniques that the supervisee finds consistent with his or her theoretical orientation to clinical practice. Then the supervisee must try out these approaches and techniques to see if they are effective and personally comfortable. The degree to which a supervisee is comfortable in using a technique is determined not only by the supervisee's experience in using the approach or technique but also by how closely the approach or technique fits into the supervisee's interpersonal relationship patterns. For example, some beginning supervisees experience discomfort in using emotionally evocative techniques, such as those associated with Gestalt psychotherapy, because the supervisees would not be likely to be evocative or confrontive in any of their interpersonal relationships.

Once this initial identification and screening of approaches and techniques is done, supervision can focus on making the supervisee more comfortable in the use of the selected approaches and techniques. In this process the supervisee learns the technique so well that it can be applied spontaneously and with confidence. As the supervisee integrates techniques with general interpersonal behavior, the supervisor expects to see more effective clinical results and a more confident and independent clinician.

Focusing on the intent of the supervisee is a characteristic of the Integration model that clearly separates it from other models of supervision. Motives of the supervisee are examined not to decide on the supervisee's degree of neuroticism but to determine his or her effect on the therapeutic interventions with the client. The supervisor is careful not to question the sincerity of the supervisee's intentions; instead, the supervisor questions and helps the supervisee to question the intent of the supervisee's interaction with a particular client. Sometimes the supervisee's intent contrasts with the message that is communicated to the client. In the case study below, Frank, the supervisee, wants the client to become more independent from her father and the destructive father-daughter interaction. Frank, however, feels almost completely responsible for the client. Audiotapes or videotapes would likely show that Frank communicates a meta-message to his client that she is not ready to be responsible and independent and that Frank will take responsibility for her—exactly the opposite of what Frank wants for her. A goal of the Integration model is to clarify supervisees' intentions, how they are communicated to clients, and the results on the clinical relationship. This clarification helps supervisees to plan any changes in their behavior that are necessary in order to become consistent with their intentions.

Although the Integration model uses existing levels of skills and personal development, the outcome of integrating these characteristics is a more effective clinician. In this model the functional relationship is collaborative, and the hierarchical distance is low. The focus is on the reciprocal interactions between supervisee and clients and could include the interchange between supervisee and supervisor and the comparison of these two sets of exchanges as described in the parallel process discussions by Mueller and Kell (1972) and by Doehrman (1976).

CASE STUDY

This case study illustrates the typical responses of a supervisor using the Integration model of supervision. The case is taken verbatim from *Styles of Supervision II*, a videotape developed by Hart (1976b) and *Instructor Manual* for the videotape written by Hart et al. (1976b). The comments in the left margin point out where the supervisor illustrates one of the dimensions of 1) the functional relationship of the supervisor and supervisee, 2) the hierarchical relationship between the supervisor and supervisee, and 3) the focus of the session.

Comments	Supervisor-Supervisee Interaction
	Supervisor: Hi, Frank. Come on in and have a seat. Supervisee: Thank you. Whew, I don't know. You have time this afternoon to talk, right? Supervisor: Right, sure. Supervisee: Well, I'm having a little trouble with a client I'm seeing, I think I talked to you about her before, her name is Janet. To refresh your memory, she's cut her wrists about three times, and she's overdosed a few times here at the school, well, not here at the school, actually, on weekends at home, and she has a, it seems like it occurs every time she has a fight with her father. And she told me about a month ago that she had had an abortion about 2 years ago. And

Comments	Supervisor-Supervisee Interaction
	it seems, well, it seemed at that point that she couldn't let her anger out at her father because she had hurt him so much. Like her parents had sat around and cried for like 2 weeks before she got the abortion and, uh, we've been working on a behavioral thing, where she would start feeling angry on a Saturday night with her father rather than going upstairs to the bedroom, she would go out to a restaurant, and kind of calm down and not get hooked into a fight or start one herself. And it went along for a . . . it went along okay for a few weeks, but this past weekend, you know, she's cut her wrists again and, I don't know, at this point I'm kind of floundering because I'm. . . .
Supervisor identifies what he believes the supervisee is feeling toward the client and his progress with her.	Supervisor: It sounds like you're pretty disappointed that all the work you put into it hasn't seemingly gotten you anywhere.
	Supervisee: Yeah, it seems like, you know, gee, am I wasting her time and my own? Am I doing something wrong, or you know, I really feel helpless. It's, what now?
Supervisor checks to see if a parallel exists between the feelings of the supervisee and the feelings of the client.	Supervisor: That's kind of a good word, because that's the one I was going to use, too. It does seem like you're feeling very helpless. It sounds as though that may be a feeling that she has too—do you think that's possible? That, kind of, there isn't any way for her to do anything with her relationship, any way to express herself, and so she kind of goes for the suicide as a last resort, almost.
	Supervisee: Yeah, yeah. And talking, well, I was talking to her just this morning and she's kind of like more depressed than I've ever seen her, because she'd been working on this, and she said her mind just went blank, and she went upstairs, and next thing you know, she woke up in the hospital. And, uh, yeah, so she's pretty well depressed, too. I don't know

Comments	Supervisor-Supervisee Interaction
	if there's a lot of that going around, or something. Supervisor: Yeah, I'm really sensing that same thing happening right here, though, that you're feeling pretty down about the whole thing. Supervisee: Yeah. I just don't know what to do next. Supervisor: I guess I'm kind of, I'm getting a feeling that maybe there's some sort of answer—that maybe I could tell you, "This is what you should do with this person at this point."
Supervisee describes the collaborative relationship between them. Supervisee accepts responsibility by telling the idea he has regarding the client.	Supervisee: Well, I know you can't really give me an answer you know, or maybe I'm hooking you into something else, maybe I'd like an opinion or something. Just somebody to bounce ideas off of. I don't know, I've been toying with the idea of, I don't know, possibly referring her out, I'm not sure whether I'd be escaping, or whether that's the wise thing to do.
Supervisor focuses on the causes of the supervisee's desire to refer the client. Supervisee responds with a fundamental concern produced by his work with this client.	Supervisor: You're referring her because you don't feel like you can deal with the situation? Supervisee: Yeah. And that takes a lot to admit. And like, you know, it's part of my work, to be able to help somebody, but to admit to myself, you know, like, "Gee, you can't help this person," or something. Supervisor: Yeah. Somehow that makes you, what, less of a. . . . Supervisee: A counselor, less of a, maybe, self-image, you know. Gees, am I in the wrong profession? Supervisor: So you're really having some serious questions about yourself? Supervisee: Yeah, because. . . . Supervisor: Of how adequate you are, I guess, in dealing with things that come up.

Comments	Supervisor-Supervisee Interaction
	Supervisee: Well, what I think, there are other cases, okay, where I'm making progress. But its the losses; it's kind of like uh, you know.
Supervisor suggests another feeling the supervisee may be having toward this particular client.	Supervisor: Yeah. There's another feeling that I have—something about you're really feeling as though you have to take on a tremendous amount of responsibility for this girl, kind of like you're her only resort, that if you can't help her, then it's a pretty helpless situation, and you're kind of a helpless person. Is that accurate?
	Supervisee: Yeah, Yeah. I'm thinking, yeah, she had mentioned that, well I talked to her mother, too, and her mother confirmed that she really didn't want to go to anybody else, and the mother didn't really want to take her to a doctor or anything. And it's kind of like, here it is, and it's on me. And I've been . . . Well, I thought I was coping with it fine, I thought we were really getting somewhere. As a matter of fact, she had been talking about the fights with the father, and the drugs, and cutting herself as past tense and everything—it was almost as like well, I was back in, you know, way before, past tense. And . . .
	Supervisor: Kind of life that was a different life then?
	Supervisee: Yeah. It was like she turned over a new leaf, and we were working on communications skills, and, I don't know, role-play—I was trying to get her interested in, you know, making suggestions, and she was going out too, like instead of staying home Saturday night, going out bowling with her girlfriends. She can't drive, she's an epileptic, she can't get a license, but she was meeting, you know, like, creating new ways of getting out.

Comments	Supervisor-Supervisee Interaction
Supervisor changes the focus from the supervisee describing the client to describing his desired behavior and optimum relationship with her.	**Supervisor:** Okay. Instead of getting back to her, let's try and center in a little more on what might be happening right now. Because I'm kind of concerned about that helpless feeling you have, and that depressed feeling, and I guess, again, tying it into the responsibility you seem to be taking for her life. And the way you present it is almost like, well, "It's on me," almost kind of like you're out of control with it, like you don't have any say in how much of that responsibility you want to take, how much . . . what kinds of limits you want to set. Is that the kind of relationship that you want to have with her?
Supervisee explores his approach with the client and how he has changed toward her.	**Supervisee:** Well, in the beginning, yeah, I was, you know, I wanted to take the responsibility, and sort of let her learn, and yet, gee, I'm even saying, "let"— that's a lot of control. Let her discover how to be responsible for herself, make decisions, get it together. And, you know, I was aware that I was doing that in the beginning, but at this point I'm still, you know. . . .
Supervisee changes from the more impersonal and external "you" to the word, "I".	Oh, at what point do you, do I stop being responsible, or stop feeling, like, can I really have control over the feeling of it, that's even more, because I'm thinking about this after I go home at night.
Supervisor checks to see if the supervisee's behavior with his client is similar to his behavior with other clients.	**Supervisor:** Right. Is this something that you're seeing kind of, your behavior is a typical kind, for other cases that you can think of, maybe with other females, or generally with other cases?
	Supervisee: Uh, I would say mostly on other females. I have noticed it, okay, I tend to think a little bit more with, when I'm working with men, it's, I'm a little bit more selfish. . . .

The supervisor in this case believed that the supervisee, Frank, had the knowledge and skill to work with this client once Frank was able to 1) control his feelings of disappointment and helplessness and 2) reduce the overprotective behavior he had been exhibiting toward the client. These two issues were identified by means of Frank's self-report and the supervisor's observation of Frank's behavior in the supervision session. The supervisor kept the session focused on Frank's behavior with the client and Frank's feelings toward their interaction. Frank saw his supervisor as a person to "bounce ideas off of" in a collaborative fashion. The supervisor's comments were intended to reduce the hierarchical distance between them.

TECHNIQUES

All supervisory techniques are designed to bring about changes in supervisees. As described in Chapters 3 and 4, some supervisors wish to have supervisees change in clinical skills, others seek changes in insight and affective sensitivity. Supervisors using the Integration model of supervision want supervisees to use their existing skills and knowledge more spontaneously and naturally by understanding the manner in which the skills and knowledge can best be used. Sometimes, as in the case study above, the supervisee may discover that his or her intended behavior differs from the behavior actually displayed toward the client and needs to be modified in future sessions. The supervisory techniques employed with the Integration model will emphasize the subtle and powerful interaction between supervisee and client. An assumption of most supervisors using the Personal Growth or Skill Development model is that client change occurs in a linear fashion; that is, the clinician's action causes a client reaction, but in the Integration model the clinician and client are seen as an interactive unit with reciprocal effects upon each other. In other models of supervision the supervisor uses techniques to 1) gather data about the supervisee upon which teaching interventions can then be made, or 2) actually convey information about appropriate clinical behavior or more understanding of typical interpersonal behavior including attitudes and feelings of the supervisee. In the Integration model the supervisor uses techniques to gain data for both the supervisor and supervisee to examine and then to jointly establish means of learning new behavior.

Self-report

As is the case in the Skill Development and Personal Growth models of supervision, in the Integration model the supervisee reports on one or more clinical sessions that have recently occurred, and may use case notes as a reminder of significant points. The supervisor helps the supervisee report on the interaction between the client and the supervisee, rather than solely on the supervisee's behavior, client dynamics or the supervisee's general interpersonal behavior. Supervisees, like everyone else, find it difficult to be good observers and report on their own behavior; but, they find it even more difficult to judge the effects of their behavior on clients and of their clients on them. Many clinicians have been surprised to learn later that what they thought was a highly therapeutic part of a session was not the part valued most by the client or judged to be so by the supervisor. Conversely, clinicians have experienced powerful emotional reactions during therapy sessions without knowing what the client said that touched off the response.

By using only self-report the supervisor gains only the supervisee's perception of the session with the client. The supervisor does gain data on the supervisee-client interaction, however, through the manner in which the supervisee described the previous interchange with the client. The congruence between the supervisee's attitudes and affect when describing the previously-held therapy session and the actual exchange that took place in that session may be very low for some supervisees yet very great, and thus useful in supervision, for other supervisees. The supervisor must view the actual therapy session to see the extent of correlation between the actual interaction with a client and the supervisee's report of that therapy session.

Role-playing

Role-playing is a more direct method of gathering data about supervisee-client interactions and so is somewhat more valid than self-report. The similarity between a role-play in supervision where the supervisee plays the clinician and the supervisor plays the client and the actual supervisee-client interaction, however, depend to a great extent on the supervisee's ability to behave in a consistent fashion from place to place. Consistency may be a characteristic that more advanced supervisees acquire as a result of increased competence, confidence in themselves, and trust in their supervisor. Although, as Mueller and Kell (1972) defined and Doehrman (1975) observed, supervisees' interactions in therapy sessions are frequently and inevitably reproduced, albeit subtly, in the supervision session regardless of the level of supervisee development.

The first step is for the supervisor to learn how the client generally behaves by having the supervisee role-play the client while the supervisor role-plays the part of a clinician or another person suggested by the supervisee (e.g., the client's boss, spouse, or friend). In this way the supervisor can see, with some degree of accuracy, how the client behaves or, at least, how the supervisee perceives the client behaving. Supervisors with a behavioral orientation are apt to accept the information gained in the role-play with little comment while supervisors with a more psychodynamic framework may wish to discuss the supervisee's perceptions of the client in detail.

Once the supervisor has some idea of how the client generally behaves, the supervisor role-plays the client and the supervisee plays the clinician. The supervisor should direct the supervisee to observe and remember significant parts of the ensuing interaction such as any specific feelings and thoughts that arise toward the client during the role-play and any behavior of the client that precipitated those thoughts and feelings. The supervisee also should note the client's reaction to the supervisee's behavior, especially if these reactions are unusual or confusing.

Following the brief role-play, usually no longer than 5 minutes, the supervisee shares whatever observations were gained during the role-play. The supervisor may also share reactions to the supervisee's portrayal. The intent of this role-play is to relate the information gained to the actual therapeutic interaction between the supervisee and the client. In the relatively safe environment of the supervision session, the supervisee may be able to identify feelings, attitudes, and overt behavior patterns not recognized while he or she was engaged in clinical sessions with the client. Of course, the supervisor also may suggest possible patterns indicated by what the supervisee said and did during the role-play. The aim is for the supervisor and supervisee to gain and share information, to discuss the significance of this information on the supervisee's functioning with the client, and to decide if more overt changes in the supervisee's behavior need to be implemented. Role-playing is applicable not only in individual supervision but also in group supervision of group therapists (Coché, 1977) and of marriage and family therapists (Kaslow, 1977).

Sitting-in

Sitting-in, observation, co-therapy, and tape recordings differ significantly from role-playing because they provide direct information for the supervisor about the actual interaction of the supervisee with a client that is not filtered through the perception of the supervisee. The key point is that the supervisor does not reject or replace the views of the supervisee but rather expands the supervisee's frame of reference to include the supervisor's views. As a data-gathering technique, sitting-in, as used in the Integration model, has serious drawbacks that observation or tape-review does not. The focus of the Integration model is on the interaction between supervisee and client, not merely the supervisee's intervention or the supervisee's reaction to client behavior. Sitting-in invariably changes the therapeutic context and thus alters the supervisee-client interaction. Even if the supervisor remains mute throughout the therapy session, the interaction is different. As a data-gathering device, sitting-in cannot yield valid data about the supervisee-client interaction and should be replaced by observation or tape-review.

Sitting-in, as a direct teaching technique, is applied most appropriately on an as-needed basis as a therapy session has developed. This as-needed implementation, termed *supervisory consultation* by Abroms (1977), is often used by supervisors applying live rather than immediate or delayed supervision as described in the reports by Montalvo (1973), Birchler (1975), and Hare-Mustin (1976). When used in live supervision or coaching, the intent of the supervisor is to disrupt the supervisee-client interaction because it is in some way ineffective or inappropriate.

Observation

The format for conducting an observation of a clinical session between a supervisee and a client in the Integration model via a one-way mirror or closed-circuit television is the same as the format used in the Skill Development and Personal Growth models. The supervisor and supervisee meet before the clinical session to determine what the supervisor will observe. During the session the supervisor will record notes and/or fill out a checklist, which is described in Chapter 3. Immediately after the session, supervisor and supervisee discuss the session.

In the Integration model the supervisor observes how smoothly and comfortably the supervisee uses techniques and whether the techniques seem to be an integral part of some theoretical orientation. Regardless of any differences in theoretical orientations between the supervisor and supervisee, supervisors using the Integration model look for interactions where the supervisee and client are in conflict or, instead, are in a highly functional interaction.

One helpful strategy is to have multiple observers who might be other staff members or students as described in Hare and Frankena (1972), Tucker et al. (1976), and Tucker and Liddle (1978). Observers can verbalize their observations during the clinical session so that the supervisor can report them to the supervisee later during supervision. Or the observers may present their observations directly to the supervisee in a group supervision session following the observed therapy session as depicted in the videotape produced by Hart and Liddle (1976). The views of additional observers serve as a validation (or invalidation) of the supervisor's observations, as well as a source of new ideas for the clinician.

Co-therapy

One of the most frequently used techniques in the Integration model is co-therapy, in which, for example, the supervisor and supervisee work with the client as a team. As an alternative, the supervisor helps two supervisees who form a team. These formats are discussed at length by McGee and Schuman (1970), Kadis and Markowitz (1972), Kaslow (1972), and Yalom (1975). Some supervisors prefer to form a co-therapy dyad with a supervisee (Rubinstein, 1964; Whitaker, 1976; Abroms, 1977) and others see more value in the supervisor working with two supervisees as co-therapists (Tucker et al., 1976). Field research of the supervisor-supervisee dyad by Rosenberg, Rubin, and Finzi (1968) and Van Atta (1969) provide illustrations of the complex interactions that occur between co-therapists, and in comprehensive training programs both formats may be differentially valuable at certain points of a supervisee's development.

One of the most important issues to explore and resolve is conflict between the co-therapists. Did each clinician perceive that both were operating in a supportive and cooperative manner? Did any feelings such as resentment or rejection appear toward each other? If the relationship between the co-therapists is not secure, then their collective effect on the client is diminished. Also important is the spontaneity and ease with which the clinicians' statements were delivered. Furthermore, what is the evaluation of each clinician regarding the effects of their statements made to the clients? Of particular importance is the intent of the clinician, the expressed statement to the clients, and the impact of the statement.

The beginning student in a training program or the beginning clinician in an agency is usually cast as a novice; therefore, a supervisor is needed to serve as a co-therapist or, more accurately, as senior therapist. After the supervisee has gained enough experience and competence, pairing with another supervisee or even a solo performance is allowed. The opposite sequence is advocated by this author so that two supervisees pair as co-therapists initially and later each pairs with a supervisor to conduct therapy with a group or family, and finally operating alone. In this sequence supervisees are expected to be competent enough to help the group or family selected for them and it is expected that the supervisees can learn just as much from each other and an outside supervisor as they can from a supervisor as co-therapist. One reason for this contention is that paired supervisees are able to function as co-equals without the degree of hierarchy between them that often inhibits the supervisee in a supervisee-supervisor dyad. One observation of such inhibition was in a supervisor-supervisee dyad during a 1½ hour couples group where the supervisee said absolutely nothing other than to greet the clients as they entered and to say good-bye as they left. Paired supervisees also have consistent roles prior to, during, and following the co-therapy experience, and no role-conflict or confusion is present. In contrast, a supervisee-supervisor dyad experiences a potentially confusing role change from the therapy session to the supervisory session that could limit the effectiveness of both supervision and therapy. The paired supervisees will gain the confidence with each other that will enable them to participate later with a supervisor as a more active and effective co-therapist.

Multiple supervisors used by Tucker et al. (1976), and Tucker and Liddle (1978) have been shown to be an effective format, especially for group supervision. Spice and Spice (1976) described a similar type of supervision, called triadic supervision, in which a supervisor and supervisee are joined in their individual session by a facilitator who helps the supervisor and supervisee communicate effectively. A videotape of this process was produced by Heckel, Malley, Scott, and Spice (1975). Just as the relationship between co-therapists is important, the relationship between co-supervisors is important. If the relationship can be an open and honest one then the benefits of mutual supervision are likely to be helpful for both the supervisees and the supervisors.

Audiotape and Videotape Recordings

Audiotaping and videotaping a supervisee's session with a client provides the supervisor and supervisee with abundant information about the supervisee's clinical interaction patterns. As in the Skill Development and Personal Growth models of supervision, the supervisor and supervisee should individually review the tape prior to the supervision session and select segments to discuss. The format of the Integration model differs, however, from that of the Skill Development and Personal Growth models in several ways.

In general, a supervisor using the Integration model gathers and uses data differently than those using other models. In the

Integration model supervisees should tape every session of a few clients so that the supervisor and supervisee can focus on the patterns that occur over time rather than the isolated view of a single session. Whenever possible, videotapes should be used instead of audiotapes because subtle cues can define the patterns of the supervisee and client interaction. Many of these cues are nonverbal and can be gained only through a visual recording. A further suggestion for format is that every taped therapy session does not have to be reviewed in the supervision session. For the supervisee to attain integration of skills and interpersonal behavior, a reflective discussion of the interaction patterns may be needed rather than an analysis of more data on the interaction patterns. Some supervisors, regardless of the model they use, overwhelm the supervisee with data and leave too little time to assimilate and integrate the information. Audiotape and videotape recordings provide an array of data that can easily overwhelm both supervisee and supervisor (Stoller, 1968). Supervisors should integrate the data at hand before accumulating additional data.

The data gained by a supervisor through tapes does not focus on supervisee intervention and client reaction as in the Skill Development model, or on cues about the general interpersonal behavior of the supervisee as in the Personal Growth model. The supervisor using the Integration model focuses on the relationship or interaction between the supervisee and client. The supervisor selects taped segments in which the supervisee and client are interacting in ways that are helpful and in ways that are in conflict. The supervisor notes when the supervisee uses clinical techniques that are consistent or inconsistent with the theoretical orientation of the supervisee, delivered awkwardly or smoothly, timed appropriately or inappropriately, or may be introduced with acceptable or unacceptable motives.

One of the most innovative uses of videotape and one that is appropriate for the Integration model is Interpersonal Process Recall (IPR), developed by Kagan et al. (1963). In this approach a trained "inquirer," usually a peer of the supervisee, observes a clinical session through a one-way mirror. The inquirer interviews the supervisee about the clinical session using the videotape of the recently completed session. This videotaped session may also be reviewed by the client and the inquirer while the supervisee observes through the one-way mirror. The inquirer asks the client to express his or her feelings about the supervisee. In another session, the inquirer meets with both supervisee and client and all three examine the videotape. Although this basic sequence is important

for Kagan and his associates, other supervisors re-order the sequence or delete one or more of the steps.

In the IPR approach, several assumptions and characteristics
of the Integration model are apparent. First, the IPR approach is
based on the assumption that people can become effective in their
application of previously learned skills even if only minimal skills
have been acquired. Second, the developers of the IPR method
(Kagan et al., 1969; Resnikoff, Kagan, & Schauble, 1970; Schauble,
1970; Kagan, 1975) see counseling as a bilateral relationship between counselor and client. Finally, the inquirer displays the characteristics of the supervisor in the Integration model with respect
to functional relationship, hierarchy, and focus. The IPR approach
uses videotape recordings within the Integration model in a highly
effective manner.

Group Work

Groups of supervisees using the Integration model are different
from the case conference and group discussion of the Skill Development model and from the growth group of the Personal Growth
model. For convenience, the members of a group using the Integration model are called a process group—not to be confused with
the term used by Coché (1977) primarily to describe growth groups.
Supervisees in a process group using the Integration model focus
on the process that occurs between a supervisee and clients. They
also engage in a process that helps supervisees integrate techniques
into their characteristic therapeutic behavior. This group may use
aids such as tape recordings and may have either a leader or be
conducted without a leader as in peer supervision. Because the
goals of the Integration model are more appropriate for advanced
students in training or clinicians in the field, the process group is
often conducted later in a training program or among experienced
practicing clinicians. Nevertheless, supervisees from the paraprofessional to the postdoctoral level of training can profit from the
Integration model used in a group setting.

In general the process group examines the data presented by
a member and shares their views about this data. All of the group
members are responsible for the goals of the Integration model.
The group offers opinions about the interaction described by the
supervisee, gives feedback and support about how the supervisee
might use techniques in a more integrated fashion, and questions
the supervisee's intentions in the interaction presented. Furthermore, as in individual supervision, the group examines and presents
their observations of how the supervisee seems to be feeling and

how the supervisee acts in the group when discussing the professional interaction.

The most significant drawback to using the group technique in any model is difficulty in keeping the group focused on the goals of the model. All too often a group member raises a concern in terms of a goal that is not part of the group's model. For example, a group member might ask for suggestions for techniques to help a client who has insomnia. An unsophisticated group could easily abandon the Integration model and give the clinician a dozen ideas for techniques without examining the clinician-client interaction, which would be consistent with the Integration model. Similarly, a group member might ask for some help with a personal problem that has come to light as a result of a clinical interaction. In this event the group might switch to the Personal Growth model of supervision or even to a therapy group approach without being aware that they had done so. How strictly the group attends to the goals of the Integration model depends on the skill of the leader and the understanding of and commitment to those goals by group members.

Peers

The use of peers in the role of supervisor and supervisee to accomplish selected educational goals for clinicians in psychiatry, social work, and psychology has had mixed research support. Peer supervision is no different from other supervisory techniques except that the supervisor is a fellow student or worker and not a faculty member or agency supervisor. For example, peer supervision in an academic training program usually consists of dyads formed among students in the same practicum class, indicating a similar level of training among them. When students have little experience as supervisees, no training as supervisors, and their levels of training are similar, the primary value of peer supervision is in the increased feelings of confidence and reduced fears of evaluation. Whether these feelings are important enough to warrant using peers who are untrained in supervision is a question for researchers.

Kendall (1972) and Wagner and Smith (1979) trained peers to be supervisors and supervisees so that they could easily implement either role. Training for supervisees and monitoring of their work as done by Wagner and Smith (1979) adds a valuable dimension to the confidence peers feel with each other in peer supervision.

A different format for peer supervision in training programs is having advanced students supervise beginning students (Davis & Arvey, 1978; Seligman, 1978). Advanced students have more clinical expertise and so can provide suggestions or conduct explorations of topics in a more effective fashion than students at the same level as the supervisees.

Feelings of trust among peers based on their perception of similarity may be diminished as modifications such as providing training in supervision and pairing advanced and beginning students are added. Feelings of trust—the major advantage of using peers in supervision—may decrease as peers perceive their roles or status to be clearly different. Of course, a developmental concept of training suggests that supervisees most need a sense of trust at the beginning of a training program; therefore, unsophisticated peers would be more helpful at this stage. Later, as students progress they might feel confident enough to learn the specific roles of supervisor and supervisee and even later can be paired with an advanced student. One of the most important questions in the use of peers is which format to use with students at what point in their development.

Peer supervision in community agencies has rarely been discussed other than by Todd and Pine (1968) and Allen (1976). Allen's (1976) description of a group of peers established for supervision is one of the few reports that shows how the members made the group supervisory rather than consultative. Participants were homogeneous in level of training and were experienced as supervisees and supervisors. Initially, the group was tentative and didactic, but as trust developed, more honest comments were presented in terms of critical feedback and self-disclosure of personal feelings. Perhaps because of their great amount of experience and advanced level of training, this group was able to use the Integration model to a great extent. The development of the Integration model may answer many of the criticisms in social work regarding the oppressiveness of extended supervision in community agencies (Kadushin, 1976). It is not recommended, however, that peers be used as the sole supervisory technique. A faculty or agency supervisor should monitor the supervisees in other ways so that effective training for the supervisee can be ensured and ethical and competent treatment for the clients of the supervisees is guaranteed.

APPLICATION OF THE INTEGRATION MODEL

The Integration model is used primarily with supervisees in community agencies and occasionally with advanced students in university training programs of various levels. Clinicians acquire skills as well as insight and affective sensitivity and eventually reach a point where they can and should focus on the goals of the Integration model. These goals for both students and the agency clinicians are 1) to integrate clinical skills with clients with typical interrelationships, 2) to apply skills with consistency and spontaneity, and 3) to develop awareness of motives and intentions for responses in professional relationships. All of these goals are important for the development of fully independent and self-evaluating clinicians.

A key issue is the appropriate time to work on these goals. For the most part training programs use either the Skill Development or the Personal Growth model, occasionally using both. Some professionals in social work and psychology believe that the goals of the Integration model should be achieved during the first few years on the job following formal training. Unfortunately, the opportunity for such in-service work does not always occur. Therefore, it is advocated here that the goals of the Integration model should be initiated during training programs and continued as a clinician begins active clinical practice.

How to use the Integration model is also important. The supervisor using the Integration model should not think of the supervisee as merely an implementer of clinical techniques or as a self-actualized relationship developer. Mahon and Altmann (1977) advocated the "self as instrument" concept based on the work in perceptual psychology as described by Combs, Richards, and Richards (1976).

> Perceptual psychology does not deny the importance of skills or techniques—rather it adds to them. It adds the integrating basis from which skills emerge. It is not the skills themselves which are important, it is the control of their use, the intentions with which they are used, and their flexibility or changeability that is so crucial (Mahon & Altmann, 1977, p. 48).

The Integration model helps the supervisee to apply basic clinical skills as well as self-insight and affective sensitivity in an integrated fashion that promotes effective professional interactions.

The supervisor who views the supervisee's professional relationships as a mutually interactive process will use various supervisory techniques to gather data indicating the parallel process that occurs between supervision and therapy. In the Skill Development model a supervisor might note the effects of the client on the supervisee's behavior in the session but for the purpose of developing a clinical strategy to assist the supervisee in affecting the client. In the Personal Growth model a supervisor might point out that the supervisee behaves very similarly with the supervisor and with certain types of clients but for the purpose of having the supervisee engage in self-examination about the pervasiveness of this tendency. In the Integration model a supervisor shows how the supervisee may be duplicating the client's feelings or problem in the supervision session or that the supervisee may be modeling the supervisor's behavior and feelings in the clinical session. Of course, supervisees sometimes display the behavior or feeling opposite from that which is displayed by the client or supervisor (Doehrman, 1976). In either case a supervisor using the Integration model wants the supervisee to be aware of the mutuality of effects of interpersonal interactions and to consider how knowledge of the supervisee's behavior can change the nature and course of the relationship.

A supervisor using the Integration model must also choose a format—live, immediate, or delayed. The Skill Development model is extremely effective with a live format, less so with immediate and probably least with the delayed method, although videotape recordings can be a powerful aid to review the session. The Personal Growth model is probably best conveyed through the delayed format because the supervisee can be more reflective, less effective by means of the immediate format, and least effective with the live method. The Integration model can be used with live, immediate, or delayed forms of supervision, but is probably most effective when used immediately following a clinical session. The supervisee can vividly remember what transpired in the session and does not feel pressure, as in live supervision, to implement the supervisor's suggested technique and obtain maximum or dramatic results. With some supervisees who experience high anxiety, supervision should be delayed for a day or two to let the anxiety abate. In immediate supervision, these supervisees often focus solely on their techniques or else rigidly examine their interpersonal faults that caused their disappointing interaction with the client. Other supervisees have great difficulty remembering or perceiving the clinical interaction using the delayed or even the immediate format, and the supervisor should consider using live supervision or perhaps videotape.

Evaluation

The Integration model has practical and theoretical aspects that some supervisors view in a critical light. First, the goals of the model are not yet clearly defined in terms of supervisee behavior nor is the achievement of these goals measured in terms of client behavior. For these reasons some supervisors prefer to use more traditional models of supervision. Another drawback is that the collaborative relationship, that is, the close psychological distance, can be threatening to supervisors; therefore, they may avoid this model. Although independence for supervisees is advocated in professional journals, some supervisors are reluctant for supervisees to attain independence, and some supervisees are hesitant to become independent. Because the Integration model fosters supervisee independence, some supervisors and supervisees may avoid it for this very reason. Perhaps the biggest roadblock to successful application of the Integration model is the fear of supervisors and supervisees to move from the familiar to the unfamiliar. Such movement can be hastened by educating supervisors in the advantages of the Integration model.

The advantages of using the Integration model include the fact that the goals are designed to help supervisees integrate and apply what they have learned in an interactive framework that goes beyond simple input-output notions. In actual practice the supervisor helps the supervisee in a more independent or colleague-like fashion, which closely approximates the world in which the student will soon function or in which the clinician on the job already functions. By promoting supervisee independence, the Integration model has fewer of the supervisor-supervisee dependence problems that occur in the Skill Development and Personal Growth models. Independence attained through a collaborative relationship helps the supervisee realize that the goals of clinical competence are more than a repertoire of clinical techniques or being insightful and sensitive. The Integration model stresses the individual responsibility of the clinician to accept the goals of the model as ongoing goals that must be maintained throughout his or her career.

SUMMARY

The Integration model is applied by supervisors (Kurpius & Baker, 1977), although the model has not been previously specified in the supervision literature in terms of goals, characteristics, or techniques. The collaborative relationship, the low hierarchical distance between supervisor and supervisee, and the focus on the supervisee's professional interaction patterns show the Integration model to be significantly different from both the Skill Development and Personal Growth models. Because the goals of the Integration model depend on supervisees' prior attainment of some level of clinical skills and personal growth, these goals are of a higher order than those of the Skill Development and Personal Growth models.

For this reason the Integration model is not in competition with other models in the way that the Skill Development and Personal Growth models are in competition with each other.

The Integration model, more than other models, is highly applicable to clinicians in agencies. Many professionals, especially in social work, have criticized bitterly the authoritarian manner in which they have been supervised on the job. The Integration model engages the supervisor and supervisee in a mutually responsible collegial relationship that values the participation of the supervisee equally with that of the supervisor. Students might also prefer this model during the later part of their program, when they have acquired a degree of confidence about their skills and level of insight and affective sensitivity. Depending on the supervisee's level of development and the supervisor's beliefs about the goals to be attained through supervision, the Integration model provides a valuable service.

Finally, supervisors of all theoretical orientations to therapy can use the Integration model. The goals of the model are ones that all clinicians can agree are valuable, although the particular techniques they use to achieve the goals may vary widely. Once these goals are accepted, supervisors need to establish the amounts of skill training and personal growth necessary for the Integration model to be implemented. Field research can be used for determining these amounts.

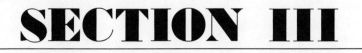

SECTION III

PRACTICE
OF CLINICAL
SUPERVISION

Chapter 6

Developmental Stages of Supervision

INTRODUCTION

The purpose of this Chapter is to describe the typical ways in which supervisees change over time during supervision, and the implication of these changes for supervisory practices. Just as developmental psychologists examine the changes in human beings as they age, so must supervisors be cognizant of the changes among supervisees as they develop. The term *developmental* implies a dynamic process that occurs over time in which supervisees acquire professional and personal behaviors and cognitions that necessitate new reactions to, new goals for, and new expectations of supervision.

The Skill Development, Personal Growth, and Integration models of supervision should not be conceived of as mutually exclusive or as implying the sole use of a particular model for a supervisee's entire supervision. The basic premise for this chapter is that the supervisor, supervisee, and context change through experience and these changes have implications for the effective practice of supervision. As a general principle, the changes in the supervisor, supervisee, and context that occur over time require that the practices carried out in supervision must also change if supervisee learning is to continue.

Several assumptions underlie the developmental process of supervision. First, the expectations by the supervisor and supervisee of supervision as a process, of each other, and of themselves are of critical importance. Extreme differences in expectations lead to disappointments and frustrations and eventually to general dissatisfaction. If such differences lead to recognizable impasses and are brought to the surface by either supervisor or supervisee, resolution is possible. Moderate and minimal differences may decline over time by movement of one person toward the other or both toward each other (Morgan, 1976). If supervisor and supervisee can identify and reduce their differences early in supervision, they will have increased the likelihood of a successful supervisory experience for both of them (Napier, 1979).

A second assumption is that after supervisees gain knowledge and confidence their goals change. For some supervisees the goal may remain the same, but the standards for attainment are increased. For example, supervisees could continually work on skill development as an overall goal. As particular skills are learned, new skills are identified for possible achievement, or minimal competence in certain skills is changed to moderate or maximal competence in these skills. Supervisees working on the goal of personal growth could establish additional areas in which they wish to grow or increase their expectations of growth in particular areas. For other supervisees, minimal competence in one goal allows them to change to a different goal. For example, supervisees might begin working on skill development and, with the confidence gained through successful acquisition of some level of competence in several skills, could switch to the personal growth goal. Conversely, supervisees who become satisfied with their level of personal growth could switch to the skill development goal. An additional possibility is that supervisees move to the goal of integration at different points in their progress. Some may wait until very late in the course of their supervision and others may work on integration at numerous points throughout the process. The reactions of supervisees to the goals they have accomplished and the formation of higher standards or establishment of new goals is the foundation of what supervisors describe as *stages of supervision.*

A third assumption is that supervision is a dialectical process between supervisor and supervisee in which each influences the other. In this mutually interactive process, both persons change as the interaction progresses. Too many conceptualizations of the longitudinal process of supervision assume that the supervisor remains consistent in behavior while the supervisee does all the changing. This view implies that the supervisor has the power to make the supervisee change but that the supervisee's responses have little effect on the supervisor. In this volume, as particularly demonstrated in this chapter, it is assumed that both supervisor and supervisee proceed through supervision as a unit, both parts of which affect the stage of supervision attained and the rate of speed at which stages are attained.

Overview

In this chapter the expectations of supervisors and supervisees toward supervision are explored in order to understand what supervisors and supervisees hope to achieve and what they realistically expect to achieve. At the beginning of supervision both supervisor and supervisee may have some hopes, albeit vague, for the process that is about to begin. These hopes or expectations may be quite different from their more realistic anticipation or expectation of what will occur in supervision. The distinction between these two aspects of expectations must be kept in mind throughout the discussion of the research. The next subsection of this chapter views supervision at the conclusion of the process, through the eyes of supervisors and supervisees themselves. Finally, changes are described that took place during the supervision process. Both supervisors and supervisees have expectations at the beginning of supervision that may or may not be met according to their assessments at the conclusion of their work together. When the expectations and evaluations are compared, changes are clearly evident. Changes in expectations have an impact on the goal to be achieved in supervision and thus the model needed.

Later in the chapter, stages of supervision are posited in a developmental framework similar to that of Littrell et al. (1979), and idiosyncratic patterns of development are described. In this chapter, supervisory tasks are described that are common to every developmental stage of supervision and are applicable to all three models of supervision and the various approaches to them.

Although the three models of supervision described in this text can be applied to supervisees at any point in their professional life, the question that remains is how a supervisor is to know which model is most appropriate for a particular supervisee at a particular time. Chapter 6 shows how each model of supervision relates to the developmental stages of supervision typically experienced by supervisees. Although one model may be appropriate for some supervisees throughout supervision, changes occur within supervision for some supervisees which would necessitate a change in the model used by the supervisor. Chapter 7 explains how the models of supervision can be applied to various modalities (individual and group) and at various times (live, immediate, delayed).

PERCEPTIONS OF SUPERVISION

Perceptions that supervisees have of their supervisors and perceptions that supervisors have of themselves are difficult to compare and interpret. For example, supervisees in a masters degree program in counseling psychology who have had no prior experience as clinicians or as supervisees may be a very different group than beginning social workers in an agency who have completed a masters degree and a year of supervised work experience. When the expectations of these two groups of supervisees are compared, there can be no assumption that the expectations come from equivalent samples. Even if groups of supervisees are similar in terms of supervised or unsupervised work experience and level and type of training, the context in which the supervision is conducted will have an effect on the expectations of supervisees. Specifically, supervisees are likely to have different expectations and evaluations of supervisors depending on the agency expectations of them, the administrative procedures of the institution (university or agency), and the client population (Napier, 1979). Finally, supervisors are different because of their level of experience (Stone, 1980) and other variables, and so their expectations must not be examined as a whole. Research on expectations regarding supervision should clearly identify the supervisors, supervisees, and context so that important differences in expectations are not blurred.

A further difficulty in interpreting the research on expectations is the definition of the term *expectations*. In some studies, expectation means how supervisees believe they will be treated by a supervisor (e.g., supervisory role), and in other studies, expectation means how supervisees want the supervisor to treat them—the difference between a belief and a desire.

The relationship between what supervisees want and/or believe they will get and what they actually receive is suggested as one determinant of both satisfaction with supervision and the amount learned. For example, a supervisee may want and expect a supervisor to be an instructor in specific skills; yet, in reality, the supervisor functions as a therapist. This supervisee could become disappointed, resistance could develop, and learning could stop. Another supervisee could want a supervisor to be an instructor, but expects a therapist. Yet another supervisee could want and/or expect the supervisor to be, at various times, either instructor or therapist. The wants and expectations in these hypothetical situations illustrate the complexity of supervisees who are beginning the supervisory process. Furthermore, supervisees' expectations could have a great impact on the supervisory process including the behavior of the supervisor and how much is learned by the supervisee, as suggested by Napier (1979). Additional research is needed to test the results of the various combinations suggested here.

Expectations of Supervision

Even though the entire issue of supervisee and supervisor expectations must be viewed in a cautious manner, some general tendencies can be suggested. Upon entry to a training program or a position at an agency, supervisees have certain expectations for themselves. In the studies by Heck (1976) and Littrell (1978), two different groups of masters degree students in counseling were found to have very similar concerns about themselves at the beginning of their supervised clinical experience. The two areas of most concern to students in both studies were learning counseling techniques and determining client needs. Of moderate concern were being adequate as counselors and knowing the counselor's role. Of least concern was whether clients liked them. Even though the results of these studies are consistent, some caution should be used about interpreting and using the results. The ranking of counselor adequacy as a moderate concern and being liked by clients as a low-level concern is in need of examination. Both of these areas are what Heck (1976) and Littrell (1978) refer to as personal concerns, rather than professional concerns (counseling techniques and counselor role) and client concerns (client needs). The lower rating of personal concerns may be attributable, in part, to the context in which the survey was conducted. One could imagine that for many supervisees, having professional concerns is more easily expressed and thought to be more acceptable to others than having personal concerns. Another point is that some beginning students who are low in personal awareness could easily block out awareness of personal concerns if they are more threatening, compared to professional or client concerns. Consequently, the results of these studies should be considered.

When taken at face value, an implication of the Heck and Littrell studies is that supervisees who are concerned about certain topics such as techniques and conceptualizing/diagnosing client needs will want these concerns to be discussed and the concern reduced in some way through supervision. The supervisor of these students is faced with their goals for supervision, which may or may not coincide with the goals thought to be important by the supervisee. When the goals of supervisor and supervisee are at odds, some accommodation must be made so that an impasse does not result.

Another area of research focuses on the expectations of supervisees regarding the role behavior of their supervisor. How will my supervisor behave toward me and what is my reciprocal role? Delaney and Moore (1966) found that beginning supervisees in a counselor training program expected their supervisor to adopt a didactic-instructive role more than either an instructive-consultative, counseling, or critique of counseling performance role. This teacher role was also expected and highly desired by Gaoni and Neumann (1974) during their residence in psychiatry. Their narrative account clearly indicates an expectation that the supervisor give "help in diagnosis, practical advice about biologic and pharmocologic treatment and guidance in his relationships with patients and their families. He [supervisee] expects advice in managing and handling his cases, theoretical explanations about symptoms, etiology, and symbolic and dynamic theory. He wants a reading list and someone to discuss it with" (Gaoni & Neumann, 1974, p. 109). These authors suggest that initial anxiety among beginning residents is typically high and is manifested in the expectation that the supervisor be the person upon whom the supervisee can rely for answers and direction. Upon reflection, however, these authors also mention that an opportunity, individually or in a group, to discuss their feelings about their experience would also have been helpful.

Hansen (1965) found that students expected their supervisor to hold them in high regard, to be moderately congruent with them, and to be low in empathic understanding and unconditional regard for them. Brammer and Wassmer (1977) interpret Hansen's finding by saying that supervisees "expected to be valued by their supervisors as good students but not particularly as persons" (p. 56). This finding is consistent with previously cited supervisees' expectations and desires for a teacher-student relationship and instructive supervisory behavior.

In summary, a doctoral student in counseling psychology reflected, "As a novice counselor I wanted someone to tell me WHAT to do and HOW to do it. I was fearful to go out on a limb alone. I was seeking direction and was eager to follow it explicitly, if not blindly" (Wolfe, personal communication).

The survey by Nelson (1978), however, showed that beginning supervisees in social work, psychiatry, and clinical and counseling psychology gave higher ratings to self-awareness as a goal of supervision than did advanced supervisees. Beginning supervisees value the goal of attaining therapeutic competence as most important but have some interest in self-awareness as well.

Apparently, supervisees have similar expectations for their supervisors and their overall supervision experience, but what are the effects when these expectations are met or not met? A study by Napier (1979) shows that interns in psychology whose expectations of the internship site are met do better at certain therapeutic skills than those whose expectations are not met. As Napier concluded, supervisee skill attainment is related to satisfaction with the supervisor and satisfaction is related to having one's expectations met. This point is also supported by the research conducted by Morgan (1976).

From the point of view of the supervisor, Walz and Roeber (1962) reported that supervisors generally expect that they will be instructive. Using several instruments with a small sample, Smith (1975) showed, however, that supervisors were distributed over a wide range of expectations of their own behavior from didactic to experiential. Little empirical research has been done on the expectations of supervisors, thus leaving a void in the supervision field. Much more has been written by supervisors on what supervisees do in supervision (reported in the stages section of this chapter) and on how supervisors and supervisees perceive and evaluate the supervisory experience they have just completed.

Evaluations of Supervision

Kadushin (1974) reported that social work supervisees in agencies judged that the supervisory approach most effective for them was at the mid-point on a continuum of existential, supervisee-centered, and didactic, task-oriented supervision. Social work supervisors, however, leaned more toward the didactic approach than did their supervisees. Of the three main sources of satisfaction reported by supervisees, two were didactic in nature: "my supervisor helps me in dealing with problems in my work with clients" and "my supervisor helps me in my development as a professional social worker" (Kadushin, 1976, pp. 126–127). Correspondingly, supervisors saw two of their three most important sources of satisfaction in supervision as didactic as well. They rated as being highly important "satisfaction in helping the supervisee grow and develop as a professional" and "satisfaction in sharing social work knowledge and skills with supervisees" (Kadushin, 1976, p. 126).

Kadushin (1976) reported, however, that 48% of the supervisees completed the incomplete sentence "If personal problems came up in my work with clients I would prefer that my supervisor . . ." with statements indicating that they wanted their supervisor to "identify the problems and help me resolve them" (p. 161). But only 30% of the supervisors preferred this response to the incomplete sentence. Kadushin (1976) concluded, "supervisees indicate a greater willingness to accept the therapeutic intrusion of the supervisor then supervisors appear willing to offer it" (p. 161).

A study by Worthington and Roehlke (1979) also examines the reactions of supervisees who have been involved in a supervisory experience. In their study, 31 supervisees rated their supervisor and their supervisory experience at the end of a semester of their masters degree program in counseling psychology. Results showed that a rating of "good" depended on a positive supervisor-supervisee relationship, a structured format being provided by the supervisor, and direct teaching of counseling skills followed by encouragement to try out these skills. An item that supervisors rated as important (but supervisees did not) was giving feedback. Worthington and Roehlke (1979) surmised, "As counselors become more experienced, they may come to value more highly receiving feedback about their counseling behavior" (p. 71).

One explanation for the difference between supervisors and supervisees regarding the value of feedback is given in the study by Bernstein and Lecomte (1979). These authors showed that negative feedback to supervisees from supervisors resulted in greater distortion, more negative content evaluation and more disagreement with the supervisor than did positive feedback. A significant element in supervisees' reaction to feedback, however, was the degree to which the supervisor's feedback was congruent with the supervisee's expectancy about the feedback. Negative outcomes are produced in situations where there is little congruence between the supervisor's feedback and the supervisee's expectancy about the feedback. The Bernstein and Lecomte (1979) study indicates the need for supervisors to assess the expectations of supervisees about supervision and about themselves.

In the Worthington and Roehlke (1979) study supervisors and supervisees also differed on which supervisory behavior was related to supervisor competence. Supervisors, but not supervisees, thought giving positive and negative feedback, confrontation, and not missing appointments were important. But supervisors viewed sharing their counseling experiences, giving literature and references about techniques, and providing initial structure during supervision as less important than supervisees did.

When both groups evaluated the supervisory behavior that was most related to the supervisee's improved counseling, discrepancies emerged again. Supervisors, more than supervisees, viewed confrontation, giving positive and negative feedback, pointing out weaknesses, being available during emergencies, and not missing appointments as important. Supervisees, more than supervisors, believed providing literature about techniques, providing structure during initial sessions, calling the supervisee by name, being available other than at regularly scheduled times, and allowing supervisees to observe or listen to audiotapes of the supervisor's counseling to be important.

The dislike of feedback by supervisees described by Worthington and Roehlke (1979) is supported by the reactions of some of the supervisees in the Nash (1975) study. She explained that "Although some students, especially beginning therapists, welcome direct advice from their supervisors, others see supervisors who tell them what to do in therapy as authoritarian, intrusive, and controlling. These students often seem to experience the supervisor's directiveness as manifest distrust of their own therapeutic competence" (Nash, 1975, p. 60). Supervisors are cautioned again to consider the covert or meta-messages that may be perceived by sensitive supervisees. These messages, although unintentional, may be deleterious to the supervisory process.

Smith (1975) assessed actual supervisor behavior according to subroles, as determined by trained raters. This study is an example of increased objectivity toward supervision and is valuable for its efforts to assess supervision in a controlled research format. Smith (1975) found that supervisors spent most of their time in supervision "helping the counselor verbalize his or the client's concerns in order to bring them into sharper focus and making recommendations to counselors as to courses of action they may follow" (p. 105). Considering the research already examined in this chapter, Smith's study supports the idea that supervisors are largely didactic in their approach.

In summary, supervisors in Smith's study first clarified the concerns of the supervisee. These concerns may have been stated in terms of knowledge or techniques regarding a client or type of client or in terms of more personal concerns of the supervisee; but, regardless of initial focus of the supervisor, the majority of supervisors moved quickly from clarifying into instructing the supervisee about what to do. Even those supervisors who identified themselves as experiential in their supervisory approach followed this clarification-instruction pattern. Because the structure of the Smith (1975) study was to examine a single supervision session using experienced supervisors and actors as supervisees, both supervisor and "supervisee" had no prior relationship and knew that this single supervision session was not part of an ongoing supervision process. Consequently, supervisors with an experiential orientation may have been reluctant to use the Personal Growth model and supervisees also may have been hesitant to disclose personal feelings to a person they had just met. Furthermore, the single supervision session may have encouraged supervisors to give recommendations rather than wait for the supervisee to come up with recommendations that might have taken several supervision sessions.

In general supervisees value, at least initially, the didactic or instructional behavior of their supervisor. Supervisors also seem to value the teacher role and the activities that focus on knowledge and skills of the supervisee about therapeutic practices with clients.

Changes over Time

In the study by Kirchner (1974) beginning supervisees (at the masters degree level) in counseling psychology expected didactic or teaching behavior from their supervisors. Although a majority of advanced supervisees (advanced masters and doctoral students) also expected a didactic role, a sizeable minority expected the supervisor to focus on the feelings and personal problems of the supervisee in addition to the supervisor-supervisee relationship. The results of this study suggest that initial expectations of what is wanted from supervisors change as supervisees become more experienced. These results are supported by Gysbers and Johnston (1965) who found that over a six-week practicum in counseling, masters degree students viewed their supervisors less as teachers and more as consultants.

A survey by Nelson (1978) of students in social work, psychiatry, and clinical and counseling psychology categorized these students into beginning and advanced groups. Nelson's beginning groups in each of the four disciplines were more experienced than the beginning supervisees in any of the studies reported in this chapter. Nelson discovered differences between "beginning" (or more appropriately intermediate) and advanced supervisees. Advanced supervisees preferred supervisory methods such as direct observation and videotape review more than less-advanced supervisees; the less advanced supervisees preferred a more "directive" supervisor and advanced supervisees preferred a more "submissive" supervisor.

One explanation for the differences between supervisor and supervisee evaluation of feedback and other supervisory behavior is that the relationship between supervisor and supervisee changes from distrust to trust. Muslin, Burstein, Gedo, and Sadow (1972) showed that as supervisor-supervisee relationships improved, the validity and reliability of the supervisee's reports about clients increased. McElhose (1973) observed that as supervision progressed, supervisor and supervisee trusted each other more and disclosed more personal thoughts and feelings toward each other. It would seem that a high level of trust is one element that would cause supervisors and supervisees to have different expectations of supervision.

The supervisor's level of experience was shown by Stone (1980) to be related to the topics the supervisor expected to address in upcoming supervision sessions. Inexperienced supervisors expressed their expectations of supervision in terms of a supervisory technique they intended to use and also in terms of facts that relate to the supervisee skills, but are not tied to any counseling theory. Experienced supervisors also expressed their expectations first in terms of a supervisory technique but second in terms of the supervisee in a more personal way. It would seem that experienced supervisors may be more able to move from the Skill Development model into the Personal Growth or Integration model more readily than inexperienced supervisors.

An indepth study was done via factor analysis by Nash (1975), who identified some supervisor behavior that could account for the changes that occur in supervisees during supervision. As described in Chapter 2, the sources of supervisory authority identified by Nash (1975) were collaborative, coercive, and professional. Collaborative authority was positively correlated with changes in supervisees toward increased self-confidence, increased self-awareness, increased sensitivity to patients, more of a sense of professional identity, increased flexibility, and a change away from theory. Coercive authority was negatively correlated with increased self-awareness and was positively correlated with a change away from psychoanalysis. Another negative correlation was found between professional authority and change away from theory. The authority used by supervisors had differential effects on the changes reported by supervisees during supervision.

The focus of the supervisor, described extensively in Chapter 2, was categorized by Nash (1975) as career-focused, relationship-focused and non-technically focused. The career-focus had a significant positive correlation with an increased sense of technical skill, more of a sense of professional identity, and had a significant negative correlation with realistic and practical goal setting in therapy. The relationship-focus had a significant positive correlation with increased self-awareness, increased sensitivity to patients and change away from the medical model. The nontechnical focus had a significant negative correlation with an increased sense of technical skill. The content on which the supervisor focuses is, as one might logically assume, a factor in the changes that occur among supervisees.

What then can be concluded from the research on the expectations and evaluations of supervision? Supervisees apparently begin their clinical work with some doubts about their therapeutic competence and wish to have a supervisor be supportive of them and directive in giving suggestions, advice, and descriptions of the supervisor's experiences in clinical work. Supervisees want supervisors who are attentive and interested in conducting supervision. Beginning supervisees do not want and indeed resent feedback that is highly critical of their work especially if this feedback is different from their own assessment of their competence.

At the same time, beginning supervisees have personal concerns such as being liked by clients, but these concerns are not examined until later in the supervisory process and sometimes are not examined at all. If personal concerns are not brought up until an adequate level of trust is established, it is likely that some supervisees will never have sufficient trust in their supervisor and consequently will never raise personal issues for consideration. In addition to or instead of this trust level explanation, some supervisees may not raise personal issues because the supervisor has clearly communicated that the goal of supervision is skill development, not personal growth, and so supervisees refrain from violating the implicit contract that the supervisor has advocated.

Reports of changes that occur as supervisees advance indicate that supervisees become less defensive and more open to threatening supervisory techniques. Reports of satisfaction with supervision, however, are dependent on the supervisee's expectations at the beginning of supervision. In general there is clear evidence that the supervisor's goals, expressed through the focus of the sessions, and the supervisor's use of authority (power) have a significant and differential impact on supervisees depending upon their anticipations of the focus and authority of the supervisor. This statement forces researchers to examine not just what happens in supervision, such as the model used, but what the supervisor and supervisee anticipated would happen. A supervisor's expectation of initially using the Skill Development model may need to be modified as supervision begins and the Personal Growth or Integration model is found to be more appropriate. A supervisee's anticipation of using only the Skill Development model also may need to be altered as the Integration or Personal Growth models become more appropriate.

As shown in this section, the expectations of both supervisor and supervisee are quite likely to change during the course of supervision although the reasons for the changes are as yet unclear. Perhaps, the supervisor's and supervisee's perceptions change specifically toward each other's role or the focus each person wants to take or the hierarchical distance between them. For example, a supervisor may first view the teacher and student roles they adopt as quite appropriate and never think of changing to different roles; however, later in supervision it may be quite helpful for the supervisor to change to a collaborator role.

STAGES

Many authors have described stages through which most supervisees pass. Historically, these descriptions have served as guidelines that other supervisors could use to chart the progress of their own supervisee. Even though the descriptive literature is not as precise as the empirical studies surveyed in the previous section, it adds a richness and meaning to the factual data that have been gathered. The description of stages described in this section begins with the opinions of authors who, although they have different conceptualizations, are, to an extent, in some agreement about the developmental stages of supervision. The developmental process is examined in this chapter in terms of the three goals of supervision associated with the models described in other chapters—acquisition of knowledge and skills about clients, personal growth, and integration of knowledge, skills, and personal growth.

Fleming (1953), in an article that is a classic in psychiatric supervision, describes the stages of imitative, corrective, and creative learning. She stated that supervisees are anxious initially and concerned about their apparent lack of skills, and so they imitate their supervisor, requesting suggestions and following them specifically. As supervisee confidence increases, the supervisor corrects inaccurate interpretations or techniques that are likely to be unsuccessful. Furthermore, the supervisor moves into the personal reactions of the supervisee toward the client and how these reactions may be contributing to therapeutic ineffectiveness. The creative learning stage is where supervisor and supervisee work on the questions the supervisee should be asking in order to improve the supervisee-client relationship.

Although Fleming's article is almost 30 years old, it provides a cogent analysis of the developmental process of supervision. One important part of this conceptualization is that supervisees' increasing confidence allows for changes in the goals of learning and changes in the supervisor's behavior to take place. With increased confidence gained through success with clients, supervisees who initially needed direct instruction on what to do with clients take more initiative in establishing treatment goals and implementing therapeutic techniques. Correspondingly, supervisees become less dependent on their supervisor for specific therapeutic interventions to be used. At the same time the supervisor can change from direct instruction to corrective feedback following a review of supervisees' work with specific clients. This corrective feedback can be focused on any one or all of the conceptualizations, the skills, or the personal feelings of supervisees. Next, the shift to Fleming's stage of creative learning indicates increased confidence and therapeutic competence by supervisees that allows them to look more carefully at their interactions with specific clients. The supervisor is more of a consultant or collaborator here in guiding supervisees' examination of themselves and their relationships with clients.

Fleming (1953) implied that the stages of imitative, corrective, and creative learning are inevitable for most supervisees. Furthermore, the message is communicated that somehow supervisors will follow the lead of supervisees in these stages and behave appropriately, thus providing successful learning for supervisees. Other authors view the developmental process as a mutual one between supervisor and supervisee and use terms that describe the roles that each person takes at different stages.

Ard (1973) described the stages of developmental supervision in terms of supervisory role and suggests the stages include preceptorship, apprenticeship, mentorship, sponsorship, and peership. Preceptorship refers to the general orientation given by the supervisor prior to the beginning of therapeutic work by the supervisees; peership refers to the relationship following the termination of formal supervision. In the middle three stages, apprenticeship describes the period in which the supervisee asks for and receives specific instruction about what to do and how to do it; mentorship suggests that the supervisor critiques the work of the supervisee and helps the supervisee in a process of self-examination, and sponsorship is a period when the supervisor is convinced of the supervisee's competence and helps to instill further confidence. These general roles and stages serve as a begining guideline for supervisors. Ard seems to concur with Fleming that stages are uniformly followed by most, if not all supervisees, but, unlike Fleming, implies that the supervisor has the major responsibility for moving the supervisee through the various stages.

With some idea of stages in mind, what specific activities should a supervisor conduct at different stages that would be helpful to supervisees and thus would facilitate their development through the stages of supervision? Hogan (1964) described levels (stages) through which supervisees pass and how supervisors should behave at each level. At the first level a supervisee is in need of advice and is likely to be imitative so the supervisor should offer "tuition"—examples of what to do, support, and training in emotional awareness. The supervisee at the second level has a "dependency-autonomy conflict," which requires that the supervisor offer support, clarify the supervisee's ambivalence, give examples of what to do and, to a lesser extent, give direct tuition regarding specific clients. Level 3 supervisees have attained a sufficient level of technical skills and confidence and now seek further self-insight and clarification of their motives. The supervisor should continue giving examples but perhaps of a more personal and affective nature. In addition, the supervisor should offer personal and professional confrontation. A fourth and final level is reached where individual supervision is collaborative in nature and peer supervision is added. The individual supervisor confronts and shares in a highly personal way while consulting regarding specific clients.

Hogan (1964) suggested that as supervisees develop, certain supervisory behavior is helpful at each stage and that the behaviors helpful at one stage are different from the behaviors that are helpful at other stages.

Several accepted beliefs can be identified from the literature surveyed thus far. First, supervisors believe that supervisees enter supervision in a dependent position and proceed through a series of difficult but successful experiences with clients with the help of a supportive supervisor. Second, supervisees and supervisors begin supervision with didactic and instructional goals and later move to more personal awareness activities, and finally to more integrative goals. Third, the role of the supervisor should be to allow the supervisee to be dependent initially, to convey knowledge and skills regarding specific clients, and to allay the anxiety a supervisee presents. Later, the supervisor should help the supervisee become more independent in their relationship and in the supervisee's work with clients and should be more confrontive and corrective about the supervisee's work at a cognitive and affective level. Finally, the hierarchical distance should be reduced to the point where they can act as consultants or collaborators regarding the supervisee's relationships with clients.

As shown by the literature surveyed here, the developmental process of supervision first contains didactic instruction by the supervisor and acquisition of case conceptualization and skill acquisition by the supervisee. The second stage is additional work on supervisee skills but now through supervisory feedback on supervisee therapeutic work. Also, the second stage includes a personal awareness emphasis. Last, some form of integration or blend of skill development and personal awareness is directed toward the supervisee's relationships with clients.

These stages have numerous implications for the goals to be established for supervisees and the techniques supervisors use to accomplish these goals. A major issue first needs to be resolved, however. At issue is to what degree this pattern of developmental stages holds true for all supervisees. Is there a significant minority of supervisees who follow divergent patterns? Finally, if certain divergent patterns do not include all of the usual stages, then what responsibility does the supervisor have to move the supervisee into the omitted stage(s)? For example, Gaoni and Neumann (1974) described, from the point of view of the supervisee, the difficult stages through which, they contend, supervisees travel: 1) the teacher-student stage, 2) apprenticeship, 3) developing the therapeutic personality, and 4) mutual consultation among equals. Of particular importance, they believe, is the developing of the therapeutic personality stage. Given the importance of this stage, what if it did not appear with some supervisees? Could the mutual consultation stage be attained without prior achievement of all of the first three stages? Or, do some supervisees remain in the teacher-student or apprenticeship stage?

The possibility that some supervisees enter and remain at an imitative learning, teacher-student, or skill development stage is apparently quite possible and of considerable concern to supervisors. Dewald (1969), Ekstein and Wallerstein (1972), Mueller and Kell (1972), and Doehrman (1976) detail the conflicts between supervisors and supervisees than can inhibit and, indeed, prevent further movement of supervisees through the stages of supervision. As described by Doehrman (1976) in psychoanalytic terms, supervisees formed intense transference reactions to their supervisors. She stated, "Each therapist, feeling threatened by the anxiety mobilized by his perceptions of his supervisor's role with him in supervision, adopted a style or role with the supervisor that reflected how he experienced his supervisor" (Doehrman, 1976, p. 72). This situation prevents supervisees from any developmental movement until some resolution of the impasse occurs.

Similarly, Mueller and Kell (1972) described numerous conflicts (impasses) between supervisor and supervisee, their causes, and ways to achieve resolution. From an interpersonal framework relying on the work of Sullivan (1953, 1956), the authors stated that conflicts arise between supervisor and supervisee as a result of anxiety of the supervisee arising from the interaction of "the client in relation to others, the client and therapist in relation to each other, and the therapist and supervisor in relation to each other" (Mueller & Kell, 1972, p. 7). These conflicts may be unseen or, if not unseen, avoided by both supervisor and supervisee but, "So long as the supervisor and therapist focus their attention solely on the client's behavior and assume that managing that source of anxiety is a sufficient goal of supervision, the process of supervision will remain didactic at best" (Mueller & Kell, 1972, p. 6). From the Mueller and Kell viewpoint the supervisee or the supervisor or both could keep the process of supervision from advancing past the beginning stage.

It seems that supervision can become stalled at the intial stage and remain there for the duration of the supervisory experience unless some intervention by supervisor or supervisee takes place. Remaining at the initial stage of supervision can be attributable not only to the interpersonal relationship difficulties of supervisor and supervisee but also to the goals of the training program or agency in which the supervision is conducted. As described in other chapters, some training programs emphasize therapeutic conceptualizations and skills, others stress the personal growth of supervisees, and most programs probably blend the two emphases to some degree. Agencies, as reported by Warnath (1977), emphasize problem-solving, not personal growth in the development of their clinicians, thus suggesting that supervisees may begin and remain at the instructive or teacher-student stage.

One pattern is that supervisees remain at the stage at which they began supervision. Because supervision most often begins with a skill development focus, most supervisees who remain at the initial stage continue to work on skill development tasks. This pattern is illustrated in Part A of Figure 4. Nash said, however, that "other students, especially more advanced therapists, are interested in examining their own feelings and feel that supervisors who do not make this an important aspect of supervision are neglecting their supervisory duties" (Nash, 1965, pp. 60–61). In this case, a supervisor might initiate supervision with a supervisee, sometimes but not always an experienced supervisee, who would remain at the level of personal awareness throughout the supervisory experience. This pattern is illustrated in Part B of Figure 4.

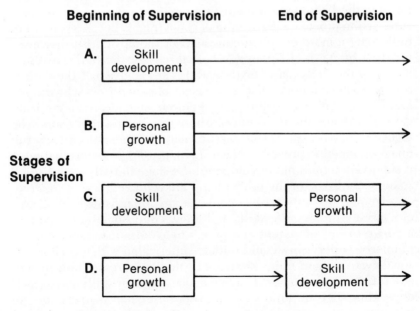

Figure 4.   Stages of supervision: alternative patterns I.

One cause for supervisees' initiating a discussion of feelings is that some beginning supervisees do not gain security by focusing on therapeutic skills and case conceptualizations because these are the very aspects of their training about which many supervisees are most anxious. One way of circumventing an examination of therapeutic concepts and skills is for supervisees to describe personal feelings and avoid discussing the client entirely.

The supervisor can also be responsible for beginning and continuing with the goal of personal growth regardless of the inclination or motivation of supervisees to move to another stage. For example, some supervisors with a client-centered approach to therapy apply this philosophy to supervision and focus only on the insight and affective sensitivity of the supervisees. Similarly, some behavioral clinicians contend that a focus on skill or knowledge acquisition is the sine qua non of supervision and focus on nothing else from the beginning through the end of supervision. To say, however, that supervisees with a phenomenological orientation should be supervised via the Personal Growth model solely or that behavioral clinicians should only be supervised by means of the Skill Development model is "simplistic" according to Brammer and Wassmer, (1977, p. 76). They continue to say that, "One can imagine the client-centered therapist undergoing a practical skills supervision process (as in the microcounseling model), just as one can imagine the behavioral therapist undergoing a personal-emotional supervision process with the aim of changing his behaviors in order to become a more effective counselor or therapist." Furthermore, research by Nash (1975) suggests that neither the Skill Development nor the Personal Growth model is as exclusive as they might sound. Nash comments that supervisees of supervisors who did not focus on acquiring techniques reported statistically significant gains in therapeutic techniques. Similarly, "even supervisors who focus exclusively on didactic issues may still promote this sort of quasi-therapeutic process" (Nash, 1975, p. 103). It seems that even if supervision does not develop past the stage initially established, some of the goals of the other stages are achieved.

To sum up, supervisees could begin supervision with a goal of attaining therapeutic skills and knowledge, some motivated by a desire to be competent and others to avoid a focus on feelings. Similarly, supervisees could initiate supervision with a goal of personal awareness in mind, some motivated to increase their insight and sensitivity and others to avoid a focus on their skills and knowledge. If neither the supervisor nor supervisee moves to change the initial goal, the pattern of supervision would be as that depicted in Figure 4, part A or B.

The typical pattern of initial stages through which supervisees pass, according to the descriptive literature in the various mental health fields, is shown in Part C of Figure 4. Here, supervisees begin working on skills and case conceptualization and later on personal growth. If supervisees should begin their supervisory experience by asking for personal growth activities and not skill development, however, an alternate pattern could develop as shown in Part D of Figure 4. In this pattern, supervisees, whatever their motivation, initially increase their personal awareness and later move into skill development activities.

Supervisees who are confident about their skills and knowledge, perhaps having had some work experience with clients prior to being supervised, may well be ready to focus on their personal development. Later, they may move into development of their skills and knowledge regarding specific clients. Sometimes these supervisees find that the skills and knowledge about which they had been confident initially have deficiencies that need to be corrected. Therefore, these supervisees find the skill development stage very valuable and quite necessary for their effective therapeutic work.

Supervisees who initially engage in a personal awareness focus because they fear showing inadequacy in skills and knowledge regarding clients may gain a sense of confidence in themselves and trust in the supervisor that allows them to turn later to the skill development stage of supervision. Some of these supervisees may even return to the personal awareness stage if they realize that their original avoidance motivation did not permit full benefit of the personal awareness stage.

The creative learning, process-focused, or integration stage of supervision, as described in this chapter, is typically found near the end of the supervisory process. A moderate level of skills and personal awareness must be achieved before these two elements can be integrated. Supervisees need the confidence that is achieved through skill development and personal awareness before they can examine the anxiety-provoking relationship between supervisee and client and between supervisee and supervisor.

The descriptive literature on supervision suggests that stages typically are ordered in the pattern illustrated in Part A of Figure 5. As stated above, however, an alternate pattern may occur; that is, supervisees begin with personal growth, proceed to skill development and then move into integration. This pattern is shown in Part B of Figure 5.

One additional variation in the sequence of stages is illustrated in Part C of Figure 5. In this sequence a supervisee works on skill development for a short time, then on personal growth for a brief

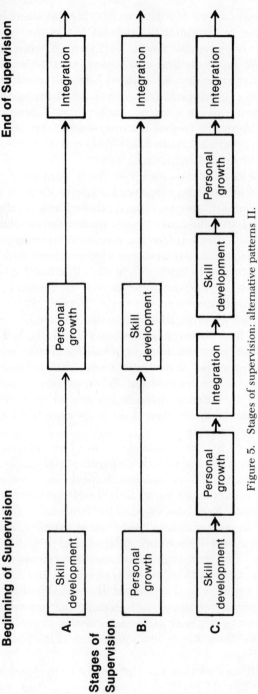

Figure 5.   Stages of supervision: alternative patterns II.

period, followed by an integration of what has been attained thus far. This cycle is repeated throughout the entire time period in which supervision is conducted. This pattern could be helpful to supervisees and supervisors who believe that the goals of skill development and personal growth are equally important and that learning can be most effective when divided into small segments. This sequence may be used by many supervisors who seem, as suggested by Liberi (1978), to focus on several goals during a single session or over several sessions.

At this point it should be mentioned that although the goals and stages of supervision may be clearly identified as shown in Figures 4 and 5, the actual behavior of supervisors in each session within each stage is not nearly so clear. Smith (1975) found that differences occurred in supervisory behavior from the first half to the second half of individual supervision sessions. Liberi (1978) also found that supervisors consistently used a particular model of supervision when instructed to do so. These studies suggest that as a supervisee progresses certain stages are reached, but overlap occurs thus causing any one supervisory session to be a combination of supervisory behavior and goals.

Research into the developmental stages of supervision conducted on larger groups than are typically studied could be helpful in determining the variation in patterns of development that occur. Once various patterns are identified, research efforts can be directed toward the degree of flexibility that supervisors should exercise in directing supervisees through various stages. For example, it is suggested that many if not most supervisees stop at a stage prior to integration, and that few proceed through this important stage. This speculation, based on informal observation of supervisees and supervisors-in-training, assumes that most supervisors in training programs and in the field are generally unaware of the typical developmental stages of supervision. Furthermore, these supervisors have one of two tendencies. The first tendency is to emphasize one initial stage (personal growth or skill development) and ignore or deemphasize the other. This tendency is based on the erroneous notion, stated in other chapters, that supervisors who have a phenomenological orientation to therapy should emphasize personal growth and those with a cognitive or behavior orientation should focus on skills to the exclusion of other goals. The alternate tendency is to form no goals and follow the lead of the supervisee completely. This allows supervisees to move quite naturally through some stages but not necessarily will they move through all stages without the direction and discussion between the supervisee and the supervisor. This tendency of supervisors is based evidently on an enormous faith in the supervisee's desire and ability to attain maximum professional development or else some unjustified restraint by the supervisor from directing and encouraging the supervisee's progress.

The position taken in this volume is that the supervisor should actively negotiate with the supervisee regarding the goals to be achieved, should suggest additional goals for the supervisee, and should encourage movement toward those additional goals. It is assumed that supervisee and supervisor, as shown in Parts C and D of Figure 4, might not reach the integration level during their supervisory experience without an effort by the supervisor. Of course, an active supervisor who moves supervisees forward can be threatening to certain supervisees, thus inhibiting their movement through supervision. The active approach, however, accompanied by support and reassurance is advocated for supervisees in general.

Supervisors must realize that with an active approach, supervisees take different amounts of time to move through the stages of supervision. Because a training program has a supervised field experience lasting from 3 months to a year or more does not mean that all supervisees can or should be expected to develop to the same level within the same time period. Training programs, agencies, and professional organizations are cooperatively developing continuing education programs for practicing clinicians (Hart, 1979). One of the assumptions of these programs is that students or interns will not develop to their fullest in a relatively brief period of preservice training and will need continued training and supervision while on the job to reach their maximum effectiveness. Continuing professional education for mental health professionals including supervision is increasing in all mental health fields (Hart, 1978b). This effort is partly motivated by clinicians who need to acquire new skills and review old ones in order to maintain their effectiveness. Another source of motivation is the increasing number of state licensure boards that require continuing education for renewal of a license to practice. These motivations lead the mental health community into a mood favorable to establishing plans for ongoing professional development.

In summary, supervision seems to proceed through distinct stages. Although descriptions by supervisors indicate that supervisees complete the stages from beginning to end in a particular sequence, there is some reason to doubt these descriptions. It is suggested that some supervisees begin at one stage and remain in it or attain only a few of the possible stages of supervision. It is also suggested that some supervisees move through the stages of supervision in a different order than do most supervisees. Only through more empirical study can the developmental process of supervision be delineated and understood.

Furthermore, the developmental concept of supervision is viewed here as a dynamic interchange in which hierarchical distance, role-relationship, and focus change over time. These dimensions of a supervisory relationship to a great extent change as the supervisor, supervisee, and context negotiate acceptable goals to be attained and the appropriate model to achieve those goals. As these goals are reached, new goals are established and thus a new model is implemented.

DEVELOPMENTAL TASKS

At every stage of the developmental process of supervision, both supervisor and supervisee have certain tasks that, when achieved, lead to the next developmental stage. When either supervisor or supervisee fails or refuses to work on a task, the supervisory dyad or group remains at that particular stage indefinitely. Consequently, supervisors who know and understand these tasks can aid the supervisee in a smooth progression from one stage of supervision to another.

The concept of developmental tasks is based on the interactional view that both supervisor and supervisee influence each other and consequently the process of supervision. It is assumed that both persons in a supervisory dyad must actively and openly participate in each task if the task is to be accomplished with maximum effectiveness. Research in supervision typically follows a simple linear model in which the supervisor's role behavior is examined and the response of the supervisee is assessed in terms of whether this role behavior was reported by the supervisee to be effective, satisfying, or in some way valuable. Conceptualizing supervisor-supervisee interaction as reciprocal in that each person is constantly affecting the other, forces new research questions and statements about developmental tasks to be posed.

The nature of the partnership between supervisor and supervisee is based on the working relationship that was established at the beginning of the supervisory process. During this time it is assumed that both persons clarified certain issues that concern supervisors and supervisees. One important issue is evaluation. Supervisees want to know how they are going to be evaluated, by whom (if not solely by the supervisor), on what criteria the evaluation is based, and what uses will be made of the evaluation at the end of supervision. Supervisees are concerned about the fairness of the supervisor and the impact of evaluations upon letters of reference, course grades, or recommendations for promotion. At the base of the concern is the supervisee's desire to be judged as competent. Concerns about evaluation can be partially alleviated by the establishment of a good working relationship but will remain a concern until supervisees begin to work on specific goals and to see how the supervisor reacts.

Another issue of concern to beginning supervisees is the amount and type of emotions they can feel free to express during supervision. During the beginning of supervision the supervisor will give spoken and unspoken guidelines to the supervisee as to how expressive to be. Guidelines that encourage emotional expression, however, must be accompanied by a considerable amount of previously established trust in the supervisor by the supervisee.

Another emotional issue that concerns supervisees at the outset of supervision is dependency. Some supervisees see the obvious potential for becoming dependent on the supervisor as an emotional and intellectual resource and fear this situation. Supervisors need to clarify their relationship with supervisees at the outset so that the fear of dependency can be reduced.

These issues are of concern to supervisees primarily at the beginning of supervision; however, they can recur at points throughout the process and should be discussed as issues in their own right, distinct from the specific topics and issues that should be discussed at the beginning of each separate stage of supervision. In the latter case the supervisor and supervisee focus on specific issues, for example, roles, techniques, and assessments that are specifically related to the goals of the particular stage under discussion, not on issues, such as evaluation, that pervade the entire supervisory process.

The developmental tasks, as described here, make the process of supervision clearer and easier to conduct effectively. The developmental tasks are 1) development of an acceptable climate between supervisor and supervisee, 2) joint-identification of a goal to be achieved, 3) joint assessment of the supervisee's level of development vis-a-vis the identified goal of supervision, 4) establishment of subgoals, 5) implementation of a supervisory technique to achieve the identified goal, and 6) joint assessment of supervisee's progress. Each of these tasks is described below in more detail so that supervisors can duplicate them with supervisees.

Climate-building

The first task is to develop an acceptable climate between supervisor and supervisee. This task includes the relationship-building that occurs at the outset of supervision but goes beyond the establishment of a good working relationship. As part of this task supervisor and supervisee examine the long-term goals that can be established and how those goals can be attained and assessed. In essence, supervisor and supervisee review their assumptions about what is important for the supervisee to learn at this particular point in the supervisee's development. In this way the supervisor begins to learn about the supervisee's perceived level of development in terms of skill development, personal growth, and integration. The supervisor also learns the future direction in which the supervisee wishes to proceed. Similarly, the supervisee learns the supervisor's beliefs about the goals that the supervisee should establish. Supervisors and supervisees often begin without clarifying their implicit objectives and roles, thus increasing the likelihood of an impasse. Attention to the long-term goals will help both supervisor and supervisee to move through short-term goals with a greater understanding of the direction and overall purpose of supervision.

Another aspect of establishing an acceptable climate between supervisor and supervisee is a discussion of the roles each person in the supervisory dyad will play in accomplishing the selected goal. For example, when referring to the Skill Development model, the supervisor would explain the teacher-student relationship and describe some typical supervisory techniques that could be used to attain the goals of skill acquisition and case conceptualization. In turn the supervisee could express interests in or concerns about the roles to be played or a technique to be used, and might suggest alternatives. In this way supervisor and supervisee function as partners in planning the learning process.

Goal Identification

After the developmental task of exploration and climate-building occurs, supervisor and supervisee must decide on a goal to be accomplished. In general this goal will correspond to a goal associated with one of the three models of supervision described in this volume. At this point the supervisor and supervisee may establish more specific subgoals if sufficient information about the supervisee's level of development is available. Otherwise, they may move to the next task in order to obtain the needed data.

Assessment of the Supervisee

The next task is to assess jointly the supervisee's level of development with respect to the selected supervisory goal. Assessment is conducted following the selection of a goal, which is in contrast to typical clinical procedures in which assessment is conducted and then goals are established to remediate the deficiencies brought to light by the assessment. In supervision each supervisee enters with certain expectations including some expectations about goals. It is suggested here that supervisees' expectations be accepted as valid until the point arrives at which other goals seem to be more appropriate. In this way the supervisee is given some respect for having already conducted some self-assessment and has established appropriate expectations.

In the assessment task, for example, if the supervisor and supervisee have agreed on skill development as a goal, then they must determine the present level of skills of the supervisee. A variety of means exist for making this determination. The supervisory pair might discuss the supervisee's work with previous clients or cases the supervisee has studied in a classroom. Or the supervisor and supervisee can role-play a clinical interview with the supervisee acting as the therapist. The supervisor can review audiotapes or videotapes of the supervisee's work or examine case notes and psychological reports the supervisee has written. The supervisor might sit in on the supervisee's current therapy sessions or have the supervisee observe and critique the supervisor's therapy session. In this way the supervisor and supervisee have some basis for establishing appropriate subgoals.

Establishment of Sub-goal

The subgoal for one supervisee might be to increase conceptualization of clients who are substance-abusers. For another supervisee, a subgoal might be to deliver effectively the previously-learned techniques of psychodrama with a group of clients. Although these two subgoals are quite different, they are still within the Skill Development model of supervision. When the general goal of personal growth or integration is selected by the supervisory dyad or group, the process of data-gathering and forming specific subgoals remains the same as that for the goal of skill development.

When the supervisory goal agreed upon is personal growth, the data collection will usually take place in discussion between supervisor and supervisee. A supervisor could also gain valuable information about the supervisee's level of personal development, however, by reviewing an autobiographical sketch of the supervisee or other personal material the supervisee has written. Review of taped therapy sessions and case notes can also be helpful. Observation of a therapy session, peer and group supervision sessions, and casual interactions with staff may also provide data for the supervisor. When sufficient data have geen gathered, subgoals can be formed. For example, a supervisee may wish to become more aware of feelings of frustration that are displayed nonverbally but not experienced internally. Another supervisee might want to understand a present response pattern of embarrasment at being complimented by others for good work. Such a particular subgoal may be only one of several subgoals that could be established under the general goal of personal growth.

Integration, like skill development and personal growth, is a general goal within which more specific subgoals can be established. The supervisor and supervisee will probably rely on the supervisee's self-report about the level of integration of clinical knowledge and skills with personal behavior. Also, observation and tape review of therapy sessions can be helpful. Then supervisor and supervisee can form subgoals such as reducing an inappropriate dependency relationship a client has formed with the supervisee.

When the subgoals have been clearly stated, both supervisor and supervisee have an equally clear understanding of what is to be accomplished. Clarity of subgoals will make assessment more precise and will reduce ambiguity in the relationship between supervisor and supervisee. It might seem that these developmental tasks of identification of a general goal, assessment of the supervisee's development, and formation of subgoals would take a long time to accomplish, especially when added to the first task of creating an appropriate climate. In practice, however, the first four steps usually take far less time than the next two and probably can be completed in one or two supervision sessions. The fact that they can be accomplished quickly in no way diminishes their importance.

Implementation of a Supervisory Technique

The next two tasks of implementing a supervisory technique and evaluating the supervisee's progress occupy most of the supervision time. The supervisory technique could be any one or a combination of techniques described in Chapters 3, 4, and 5. In general, a supervisor chooses techniques depending on the competence of the supervisee as well as the supervisee's anxiety level. As a supervisee gains competence and confidence the supervisor can use techniques that are more sophisticated and more threatening.

Assessment of Supervisee Progress

Simultaneous with the implementation of a supervisory technique, both supervisor and supervisee are informally assessing the supervisee's behavior. Such an ongoing and often unverbalized process is inevitable. For maximum benefit these separate assessments should be verbalized so that each person knows the other's viewpoint. Discussion about the supervisee's development does not have to be formal in the sense of being based on objective rating scales or being presented to each other in written form or being reported to other persons within the university or agency. A formal evaluation of a supervisee's progress conducted at the end of the entire supervisory process should be based on a collection of objective and subjective data, should be written, and should be available to immediate administrators of the university or agency. The informal and ongoing assessment should be conducted frequently so that the supervisor can modify supervisory techniques to be used and the supervisee can benefit from the reactions of the supervisor. Ongoing assessment of the supervisee's development helps both supervisor and supervisee know when the subgoals have been achieved thus allowing new subgoals to be formed or a new stage of supervision to be considered.

Concurrently, another assessment is going on, whether verbalized or not, regarding the supervisor's supervisory techniques and personal manner. The supervisor and supervisee should discuss these issues and their effect on the learning process. For example, if a supervisee believes that a certain supervisory technique or a supervisor's hypothesis about a client (or about the supervisee) is inappropriate, then this belief should be discussed. Conversely, if the supervisor believes a particular supervisory technique is proving to be ineffective, then this belief should also be discussed with the supervisee in order to determine the reasons for the failure of the technique. This procedure will help the supervisor to select a different technique. Of course, both supervisor and supervisee should discuss the positive outcomes of the learning process as well as the negative outcomes. Throughout this assessment of the learning process, both supervisor and supervisee are viewed as mutually responsible for the supervisee's progress and the effectiveness of the supervisory techniques.

In this chapter the review of descriptive literature on the developmental process of supervision concluded that many supervisees begin working on the general goal of skill development, then move into personal growth and conclude with some type of integration, while others follow a different sequence of stages. It should be made clear that, regardless of the number and sequence of the stages of supervision, all six developmental tasks described in this section apply to each stage in the developmental process. After initially establishing a good working relationship, both supervisor and supervisee should begin the developmental tasks whether they begin to work on the overall goal of skill development or personal growth. At the conclusion of the first stage of the developmental process, supervisor and supervisee should again take up the developmental tasks as a way of leading into the second developmental stage. Supervisor and supervisee would again repeat these tasks when beginning a third developmental stage of supervision. Application of the six developmental tasks to each stage of supervision shows that the entire process can be conceptualized as orderly and researchable, not random and mysterious.

Typical research studies overlook or ignore developmental stages and developmental tasks of supervision as variables. As a consequence most assessments of the reaction of supervisees to supervision are global and yield information that is difficult to interpret. It is helpful if assessments of supervisees are made in relation to specific supervisory behavior and close to the time the behavior occurred in supervision. Still, an analysis of a single supervision session can not be generalized to the entire process of supervision without considering the stage of supervision from which the single session was taken. Furthermore, it is vital to the development of the practice of supervision to conduct extensive field research and not be lured into laboratory studies that are able to be controlled in the finest classical tradition. Field studies will give greater information about the actual patterns of the development of supervision. Increasingly sophisticated methodology such as the time-sample approach used by Napier (1979) relies on increasingly sophisticated theoretical views about the developmental stages and developmental tasks of supervision. Theory and research must complement each other in an effort to raise the understanding and practice of clinical supervision to levels commensurate with standards of a mature profession.

In summary, developmental tasks are the outline that can lead supervisors to effective learning for their supervisees. When this outline is followed, both supervisor and supervisee have a clear direction in mind and so can focus on the learning objective at hand. By conceptualizing supervision as a series of developmental tasks, each relying on the successful completion of its predecessor, the supervision process becomes more teachable and more learnable.

SUMMARY

As derived from developmental psychology and their observation of changes that occur as human beings grow, the process of clinical supervision also follows discrete patterns. Most supervisees, according to descriptions in mental health literature, enter supervision with certain expectations and desires for the learning process. Similarly, supervisors have expectations about what will take place in supervision. These expectations may be realistic or fanciful, similar or dissimilar but they will have an effect on the beginning of supervision that can lead to a smooth and confident beginning or an impasse. The supervisor is urged to consider expectations as a topic to be discussed with the supervisee as much as topics such as evaluation or the degree to which feelings can be expressed. It is also important for supervisors to understand that expectations change over time as a result of experience and, like other facets of supervision, changes in expectations must be constantly reassessed.

A further point regarding change is that supervisees, in general, change in fairly predictable ways. Supervisees typically want didactic instruction and support at the outset of supervision and later ask for feedback regarding professional and personal issues, finally moving into an integration period. These changes have been conceptualized here as stages that correspond to the models of supervision—Skill Development, Personal Growth, and Integration; however, several alternate patterns probably exist as well. Supervisors who are aware of the stages and the value of supervisee movement through them are advised to use the model of supervision most appropriate for the supervisee's stage of development.

In order to carry out a particular model at a certain stage of supervisee development, supervisors can use the outline described here as developmental tasks. These tasks include: climate-building, goal identification, assessment, establishment of subgoals, and evaluation of progress. These tasks are the essential elements that should be carried out during each stage of development.

The description of supervision as an evolutionary process that changes as supervisory pairs or groups progress is made clearer by the explication of typical stages and developmental tasks. Further investigation will help to make this dynamic process one in which supervisors have an increasing awareness of how they can make this process a significant learning experience for their supervisees.

Chapter 7

Implementing Supervision

Throughout this text supervision is presented as an ongoing educational process that evolves as a result of the forces exerted by the supervisor, the supervisee, and the context in which supervision is conducted. For purposes of examination various models of supervision and developmental tasks have been separated from the process as a whole and described as isolated entitities. Models and developmental tasks, however, are integral to the ongoing and evolving supervision process. The complexity of this process is seen in that a supervisor's decisions are made not by merely plugging in a few bits of information into a general formula but rather by weighing hundreds of subtle cues from the supervisee and the context and the supervisor's own expectations based on prior training and experience. One goal of this chapter is to provide a basis on which supervisors can select a model, a modality by which supervision can be delivered (individual, group, or peer), and a temporal dimension (delayed, immediate or live) in which the model and modality are applied. During the process of supervision, as in all interactions between persons, conflicts can occur and must be resolved. Part of this chapter is devoted to delineating types of conflicts that arise and how they may be resolved successfully. Conflict resolution is an important component in the training of supervisors. Also in the chapter is a statement of goals that forms the basis of minimal supervisory competence in any of the various settings in which clinical supervision is conducted. How these goals can be structured into a training program for supervisors is also described. The final section of this chapter describes directions for future research on supervision.

CHOOSING A MODEL

The choice of a model is not a decision that is free of overt and covert influences. A supervisor's choice of a model is dependent upon the supervisor, the supervisee, and the context. These sources of influence serve to restrict the range of freedom of the supervisor but not totally confine the supervisor. In this section the supervisor is placed in the position of having to assess the characteristics of supervisor, supervisee, and context in order to determine the most appropriate model of supervision at any given time. With knowledge of these influences, supervisors may make more appropriate choices of the models of supervision. It is important to remember that because of the evolutionary nature of supervision this assessment and decision-making procedure is conducted repeatedly. Because the supervisor and supervisee change in their levels of experience, both will find that supervision must also change if it is to be a significant interaction for them. Similarly, the context in which supervision is conducted can change through, for example, the addition of new staff members and new policies, thereby influencing supervision. Decisions made by a supervisor at any given point in time must be thought of as temporary rather than permanent if supervision is to proceed with minimal conflict and maximum learning.

Supervisor Characteristics

Supervisors decide on a model of supervision to use with a particular supervisee for a number of reasons. The most frequent reason, although not necessarily a sound one, is that a *supervisor is most familiar with one particular model*—usually the one used by his or her own supervisor. Training in supervision can include all three models, but too often supervisors know of only one model. In order to give supervisors more options they should be trained in all models of supervision and then ask themselves "What model is most appropriate for me to use with this supervisee at this point in time considering this particular supervisee's level of development and the context in which supervision is being conducted?"

Another reason for a supervisor's choosing a particular model is that *a particular model may be less anxiety-producing for the supervisor than other models.* Using an unfamiliar model would be anxiety-provoking, but even if a supervisor is aware of all three models, implementing a particular one may be uncomfortable. One doctoral student learning to be a supervisor had great difficulty in using the Skill Development model because, as was later discovered, he had serious doubts about his own competence as a therapist. To him the Skill Development model meant that he had to have excellent clinical skills and "all the answers." For other supervisors the nature of the Personal Growth model, and, to a lesser extent, the Integration model examine the feelings of the supervisee, and for some supervisors this examination is anxiety-producing. Another doctoral student-supervisor used the Skill Development model as a way to avoid the feelings that would have been expressed by the supervisee if the Personal Growth or Integration models had been implemented. Through supervised training in supervision, clinicians learning to be supervisors may become aware of their affective reactions and become less likely to choose a supervision model to avoid their anxiety.

Another cause for supervisor anxiety when working with a particular model is that *the model chosen may be threatening to the supervisee* thus resulting in overt conflict that the supervisor would prefer to avoid. For example, a supervisor and supervisee who are beginning the supervisory process may both realize that the low level of the supervisee's skills and the demands of the particular client population strongly suggest the use of the Skill Development model. The supervisee, however, may be anxious about an examination of skills and may prefer to work on personal growth areas. The supervisor might then implement the Personal Growth model not because it is the most appropriate but because it arouses the least conflict and concomitant anxiety within the supervisor.

One further reason for some supervisors' choosing a particular model, in addition to lack of familiarity with models and anxiety, is their desire to choose a model that seems to be consistent with their theory of psychotherapy. This desire is reasonable; however, the supervisor's therapeutic orientation need be consistent only with the techniques and strategies used within each model rather than the model itself. Therapists of all orientations can use any and all of the models depending on the supervisee and the context.

Consistency should be maintained between therapeutic orientation and the suggestions given, the techniques used, and the philosophies espoused within any model of supervision. For example, a supervisor with a phenomenological orientation to therapy could choose the Skill Development model and make the techniques, discussions, and suggestions for therapeutic interventions to be made by the supervisee consistent with the phenomenological orientation. If this same supervisor chose to work within the Personal Growth or Integration model, the phenomenological orientation would be shown here too in the techniques, discussions, and suggestions. Similarly, a cognitive supervisor could adopt any model and then use the techniques, terms, and suggestions that are consistent with the cognitive position.

For supervisors to use only one model that seems to be most consistent with their theory of therapy is to focus on only one aspect of a supervisee's development. This singular approach is seen in the area of child development where many experts focus on one aspect of the child—classroom teachers focus on intellectual development, physical education teachers center on physical development, religious instructors focus on moral development, and parents emphasize social development. In most clinical settings where only one supervisor is usually available for each supervisee, the supervisor must be responsible for helping the supervisee to move through all stages of the supervision process and to attain the diverse goals of skill development, personal growth, and integration.

Supervisee Characteristics

The supervisor must consider a number of supervisee characteristics that influence the appropriateness of the choice of a model
of supervision. One characteristic is the supervisee's expectations
about what is to be learned. Research indicates that supervisees
generally expect to learn therapeutic techniques and knowledge
of client behavior at the outset of supervision. Later in supervision,
supervisees frequently want to develop themselves in a more personal way, and finally they wish to integrate their personal and
professional learnings. If the expectations of the supervisor and
perhaps also of the agency or training program differ from those of
the supervisee, then a conflict is present.

Another supervisee characteristic that affects the choice of a
supervisory model are the levels of supervisee skills and personal
development upon entry into supervision. These levels are assessed by the supervisor against some predetermined levels of acceptable skill and personal development. Thus, the main focus of
supervision becomes the area of deficiency. For example, one supervisee might be deficient in skills and at an adequate level of
personal development, thus suggesting to the supervisor that the
Skill Development model might be used. In another case, a supervisee might enter with a high level of skills but with a less than
adequate level of personal development, thereby prompting the
Personal Growth model. Assessment of the supervisee, although
done throughout supervision, is particularly important at the beginning of the process.

Supervisors should be aware that some supervisees will have
been supervised previously in their place of work or in courses
they have taken, thus affecting their expectations for and feelings
about the upcoming supervision sessions. If prior supervision was
satisfactory, the supervisee's expectations will be positive. If the
supervisory experience had been negative, the present supervisor
must overcome this mental set. In a similar vein, a supervisee with
prior supervised experience may be comfortable with a particular
model, set of techniques, modality, or form of temporal application
and may expect the present supervisor to follow the same pattern.
In one case the supervisee had been supervised with a focus on
the skill acquisition goal of the Skill Development model through
group supervision in a live supervision format supplemented by
individual supervision where videotapes were critiqued. Her new
supervisor expected to use individual supervision with only the
self-report technique in a delayed format and the case conceptual-

ization goal of the Skill Development model. Needless to say, lengthy discussions were necessary before supervision was arranged in a form that was acceptable for both of them.

Context Characteristics

The context in which supervision is conducted has been largely ignored by researchers and theorists even though social scientists such as Bateson (1979) have long emphasized the influence of context on human interactions. Apparently, most researchers believe that the influence of the supervisor overshadows the influence of either the supervisee or the context. It is assumed throughout this text, however, that the context can have an impact that is equivalent to that of the other two components of the supervisory process. For example, the faculty in a training program could agree that skill development is the primary goal that students should work to attain while in the program. Consequently, subtle but significant pressure would influence both supervisor and supervisee to adopt the Skill Development model of supervision. Pressure of this sort exists in all settings and must be identified if supervisors are to make a more independent choice of a model of supervision.

Some of the sources of contextual influence on supervisors are assessment criteria for supervisees, characteristics of the training program or agency, such as the dominant theory of training, the time allotted for each supervisee, the number and type of clients assigned to each supervisee, and the criteria by which the supervisor is evaluated. These characteristics, discussed below, define to an extent the goals that can be reasonably accomplished and thus the model of supervision.

One of the most obvious sources of influence is the criteria used in formal assessments of supervisees in the agency or institution. For example, students or staff members may be assessed by a written examination indicative of knowledge acquisition or case conceptualization, or by supervisor rating sheets and reports containing items aimed at personal growth or integration. The emphasis incorporated in such an assessment procedure conveys an unspoken message to supervisors that a certain goal is more important than others and that supervisees' failure to meet that goal may result in negative evaluations, no salary increase, or dismissal. An assessment system that contains multiple criteria and data-gathering techniques suggests that supervisors are expected to help supervisees attain several goals, thereby suggesting the use of more than one model of supervision. Regardless of the number or quality of assessment criteria used, these criteria are an obvious example of a source of influence within a context.

The theory of training of a program or agency although frequently not articulated specifically, may be conceptualized in terms of the goals supervisees should attain being somewhere on a continuum from theoretical to pragmatic. Training programs are frequently more theoretical than agencies because training programs prepare clinicians with skills that are applicable to a variety of clients and in numerous types of settings. Agencies, however, want clinicians to learn the skills that are specifically useful with a particular population and in a particular setting. This difference between training program and agency suggests that supervisors in an agency may be influenced to use the Skill Development model and focus on the skill acquisition goal rather than other models and goals. Conversely, supervisors in training programs may feel more free to use several models rather than or in addition to the Skill Development model only.

Another pressure of the context on supervisors is the time allotted by the administration for supervision. If a supervisor has a large number of therapy cases and administrative duties in addition to a large number of supervisees, then supervision is not likely to be the primary task of the supervisor. It seems that the effects of supervision are measured in less visible ways than other duties performed by supervisors. Administrative competence is evaluated typically by how long a person takes to complete assigned tasks, the length and thoroughness of reports, and involvement in administrative planning sessions. Clinical competence is measured commonly by the amount of client contact per week, number of cases closed, groups conducted or rate of recidivism. These measures of administrative and clinical competence may not be adequate, but they are visible compared to any measures developed to assess supervisory competence. Consequently, supervision becomes an area that is examined less closely by administrators in training programs and agencies, thus implying to faculty or staff that supervision is not as important as other tasks. Ultimately, when busy schedules of faculty or staff demand that certain functions be slighted, supervision frequently is the first on the list.

Busy schedules also affect the type of supervision, that is, administrative or clinical, that is delivered. When a supervisor has a variety of duties and too little time for supervision, the clinical aspects of supervision are likely to decrease in favor of the administrative aspects. Under the pressure of a busy schedule, supervisors may move into a case management approach in which they briefly review all or most of the supervisee's clients and their progress rather than focus on the learning of specific objectives with several selected clients. In the more administrative case management approach, supervisors can be more assured that supervisees are making no major errors with any client; but, of course, the supervisees may be making minor errors with all of the clients that go undetected. Furthermore, this approach never raises the level of competence of the supervisee.

Under the pressure of time, skill acquisition and case conceptualization goals are likely to be emphasized in lieu of personal growth and integration goals that require a more thoughtful and less time-constrained context. A supervisor with less time-pressure and few supervisees has more freedom to explore new techniques and combine various techniques in order to help the supervisee move through the supervision process.

Closely related to the issue of time allotted for supervision are the number and type of clients seen by the supervisees. In a training program the primary purpose of the students' working with clients is to improve the professional competence of the students; however, the primary emphasis in agencies is on effective and efficient delivery of service to the community at large and to specific clients. In either training program or community agency the number and type of clients of the supervisee affects the choice of a model of supervision. If the number of clients per supervisee is large then the supervisee may feel pressure to keep the supervisor at least minimally informed about most, if not all, of the clients. In the minds of some supervisees the informed supervisor shares in the responsibility for the clients' welfare and so will intervene in those cases where the supervisee has erred by omission or commission. This posture sacrifices depth for breadth and defeats the purpose of clinical supervision.

Furthermore, the pressure of a large number of clients, especially on a beginning clinician, often leads to a supervisee's request that the supervisor provide specific interpretations of the clients' problems and give definitive suggestions as to techniques to be implemented with each client. This request influences the supervisor toward using the Skill Development model that includes the goals of understanding client behavior and developing supervisee techniques.

In a similar way the type of clients seen by supervisees creates pressure on supervisors. Supervisees working with particularly difficult cases, perhaps those with a poor prognosis for change, may experience high amounts of frustration and feelings of incompetence. These feelings could lead to a request for the supervisor to provide techniques to be used, thus prompting the supervisor to use the Skill Development model of supervision. Or, the supervisee could be prompted to examine the feelings of frustration and incompetence as personal issues that must be understood as part of personal development. In this case the supervisor may decide to implement the Personal Growth model of supervision. In some agencies and training programs beginning clinicians are assigned cases that are of a less severe nature, for example, acute rather than chronic, neurotic rather than psychotic, outpatient rather than inpatient, or functional rather than dysfunctional. In this way supervisees can develop on a gradual basis from the cases requiring minimal skills, personal development, and integration to the cases requiring maximum development of these characteristics.

Finally, the criteria on which supervisors are evaluated influence their choice of supervisory model, even though formal evaluation of supervisors is usually nonexistent. For example, in some agencies supervisors are evaluated on the number of cases accepted and subsequently terminated by their supervisees or by the supervisor's knowledge of the supervisees' cases. These criteria press the supervisor to review all of the supervisees' cases and to conduct didactic supervision that will help the supervisees move clients quickly through the agency. There is no qualitative assessment of the supervisor's effectiveness with supervisees. These criteria and the other influences of the context impinge on the supervisor's choice of a model of supervision.

Contextual influences do not function in isolation but combine to form pressures on supervisors that are difficult to separate into clearly identifiable units. For example, the number and type of clients seen by a supervisee is one combination of characteristics that interacts at a simple level. A supervisee may be assigned a large number of very difficult clients, which may lead the supervisee to request the supervisor for brief conceptualizations and techniques in order to stay in control of these clients. In contrast, a supervisee in a different training program or agency may be assigned a relatively low number of clients who are not so difficult. In that instance the supervisor may experience more freedom in choosing a model, might apply more than one model as supervision progresses, and could try a variety of supervisory modalities and temporal application of models that are appropriately suited for the supervisee. These contextual influences are shaped by one issue more than any other—the agency or training program's position on the training–service delivery continuum.

The development of the philosophy of the training program or agency regarding the balance between training and service delivery cannot be left to chance. Faculty or staff members must decide on the degree of their commitment to training as counterposed with the realistic obligation to provide service to the community. Obviously, a training program has its primary emphasis on training; but it cannot relinquish its responsibility to help supervisees deliver the most effective service possible during their learning experience. Similarly, an agency has service delivery as its main concern; but it cannot let this concern eliminate the efforts of supervisors to provide ongoing development for supervisees. Once a philosophical position has been determined, specific procedures reflecting this position can be established in terms of issues such as numbers and types of clients for supervisees.

In summary, the process of clinical supervision is influenced by various characteristics of the supervisor, the supervisee, and the context in which supervision takes place. The main characteristics of the supervisor include the familiarity of the supervisor with a particular model, anxiety produced by a particular model, and/or a desire to be consistent with one's theory of psychotherapy. Supervisee characteristics influencing supervision are their expectations of what is to be learned, levels of supervisee skill and personal development, and previous supervisory experiences. The characteristics of the context examined here were the criteria by which the supervisee and supervisor are evaluated, the dominant theory of training, the time allotted for supervision, and the number and type of clients assigned to each supervisee. All of the characteristics of the supervisor, supervisee, and context interact in a complex manner often resulting in conflicts that must be negotiated openly so that the supervisory process may take place with maximum opportunity for supervisee development. With some knowledge of these characteristics the supervisor may be better able to establish a workable plan by which effective supervisee learning will take place.

USING SEVERAL MODELS OVER TIME

Although some supervisors believe that skill development is the primary goal that should be attained by supervisees, other supervisors believe that personal growth is the primary goal. Most supervisors probably believe that both of these goals should be attained as well as the goal of integration. As defined in this text each of these goals is aligned with one of three separate models of supervision; therefore, if all three goals are to be accomplished then all three models of supervision must be used sometime during the supervisory process. As described in Chapter 6, supervisees typically request certain experiences at various points during supervision. This fact coupled with the preferences of supervisors and the pressures from the context for certain goals make the use of several models seem quite appropriate and probably inevitable. The purpose of this section is to indicate the typical pattern of supervisors, which is to use several different models within a particular session and over time, and also to demonstrate that the planned use of several models throughout the process is beneficial to the supervisee's development.

As Bernard (1979) stated, counselors should be trained in all of three skill areas that she labels as 1) process (e.g., using reflection, confrontation, etc.), 2) conceptualization (e.g., becoming comfortable with feelings, attitudes, and values), and 3) personalization. By achieving some acceptable level of development in all three areas, an overall level of professional competence is assured. But how discretely are these functions attained in actual supervision sessions?

Research by Liberi (1978) showed that supervisors were able to apply a single model of supervision quite consistently when told to do so. This same study suggests, however, that supervisors needed an occasional corrective comment when they varied, knowingly or unknowingly, from the model they were to implement. The scale developed by Hart (1979b) is used to categorize the model(s) used by supervisors with actual supervisees. The content analyses done by Hart (1979b) showed that in a single supervision session several models are used, although one model is typically used more often than either of the other two models. Previous assumptions about the consistency of models used are now called into question. Research by Smith (1975) suggested that supervisors were very similar to each other in their communication patterns during a single supervisory session but may have varied widely in the focus of their communication. It seems more likely that Smith's (1975) supervisors spent time in all of the models of supervision (varying the content) but expressed themselves in a similar fashion regarding the various contents, that is, clarification of supervisee statement and suggestion of techniques.

How uncomfortable the change from one model to another depends, in part, on how thoroughly and how clearly the supervisor and supervisee discuss the change from the goal at which they are presently working to a new goal, thus another model. Some supervisors may conduct thoughtful and open discussions with supervisees about new goals and other supervisors may move abruptly into the new model with no warning or agreement. In order to make supervision maximally effective supervisees must understand the process, the goals, and the direction in which they are moving. Therefore, it is advised that supervisors undertake the developmental tasks described in the previous chapter that allow the supervisee to move from one goal to the next in an informed and motivated manner.

As illustrated in Figure 6 a supervisor at first might vary from model to model, but probably will soon settle on one model for a period of time, then another model. Finally, as the supervisee's skills and personal awareness increase to sufficient levels, the supervisor may direct supervision into the Integration model. Of course, the pattern shown in Figure 6 is not followed by all supervisors but is probably typical for many supervisors. The validity of this pattern is supported by the developmental sequence outlined by Littrell et al. (1979).

Fleming and Benedek (1966) described the changes in the emphases within a single supervision session by saying, "There is a constant oscillation between experiencing and observing the experience, between empathy, introspection and insightful choices for technical action, and between analyzing his [the supervisee's]

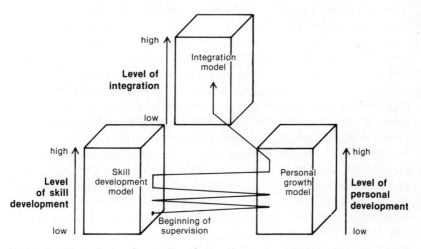

Figure 6.   Typical use of several models with a supervisee throughout the supervisory process.

patient and himself in an effort to correct his mistakes and develop creative skill in his professional work (p. 32)." The oscillation that occurs at the beginning of supervision reflects the negotiation that occurs between supervisor and supervisee. It is probably a testing mechanism by which supervisor and supervisee decide on a model to implement for a longer period of time.

Supervisors are advised to remain sensitive and flexible so that they are aware of the various goals requested by the supervisee and the model favored by the context. Also, supervisors should be alert to the changes in goals that can and should occur as supervisees progress through the developmental process of supervision so that appropriate goals are achieved according to the particular characteristics of the supervisor, supervisee, context, and developmental stage of the supervision process.

CHOOSING A MODALITY

A supervisor chooses not only a model but also a modality (individual, group, or peer) by which the model is applied. As discussed in Chapters 3, 4, and 5, modalities have different effects and should be chosen with these effects in mind. This section contains guidelines for using the various modalities and a description of the various combinations of modalities and model.

Modalities

Any of the three models of supervision described in this text may be applied via the individual, group, or peer modality. Each modality has certain strengths and weaknesses that are brought out in the implementation of a particular model. In general the rule followed throughout this text is to begin at the least complex level and proceed gradually to more complex levels. When applied to modality, this rule suggests that supervisors begin with individual supervision and later add group and/or peer supervision. Individual supervision is seen as the least complex, followed by group supervision as more complex and then peer supervision as most complex. Supervisees, especially those with no prior supervision, will be most familiar with the one-to-one format, and so individual supervision should be used initially. Many supervisees have had no experience as members of therapy or growth groups and no experience as participants in peer-led dyads or groups. Consequently, starting out with group or peer supervision could be quite difficult for these supervisees. Supervisees need to learn the appropriate roles for effective group and peer interactions (in dyads or groups) before being placed in a group or peer learning situation with such a specialized focus. Those supervisees who do not know the appropriate roles will not only fail to achieve the goals of supervision but also will prevent others from achieving these goals. Beginning with individual supervision allows supervisees to gain confidence about themselves and to understand the overall purposes of supervision before moving into more complex modalities.

A second principle is to avoid supervisee overload. In a society where "more" is synonomous with "better," supervisors sometimes combine all three modalities to achieve maximum learning for supervisees. As described in the discussion of the developmental nature of supervision, supervisees need some time to reflect on their clients and on themselves, and so all three modalities used on a weekly basis may overload the supervisees resulting in diminishing returns. Quite simply, supervisees can feel more anxious about their performance in the various learning situations than in learning itself. Although some supervisees function quite well under these demands, supervisors should be alert to those who are not yet ready to engage in this demanding environment.

A further rule is to use modalities selectively rather than interchangeably. Some supervisors who enjoy and are successful at conducting therapy groups often use the group modality exclusively or with individual supervision as a supplement (see pattern A in Table 1). Other supervisors use individual supervision for the initial period and then switch to group and peer supervision (see pattern B of Table 1), often for the main purpose of reducing the total time per week they must allocate to conduct supervision. Unfortunately, the modalities are not wholly interchangeable and should not be used in place of each other for reasons such as administrative efficiency. It is advised that individual supervision (see pattern C, D, and E in Table 1) be used as the primary modality. Supervisors may reduce the frequency with which individual supervision is conducted (see patterns F and G of Table 1), but should never replace individual supervision totally. If the relationship between supervisor and supervisee is as important as the literature suggests then individual supervision should be maintained as the primary modality of supervision.

Once a pattern of individual supervision is established supervisors must decide on the value of adding group and/or peer supervision. Group supervision offers a broad spectrum of opinions and examples thus increasing the breadth of input a supervisee receives compared to individual supervision. Group supervision is particularly valuable when each supervisee works with only a few

Table 1. Patterns of modalities of supervision

Pattern	Week 1	Week 2	Week 3	Week 4	Week 5
A	Group; individual	Group	Group; individual	Group	Group; individual
B	Individual	Individual	Individual	Group	Group
C	Individual; group	Individual; peer dyads	Individual; group	Individual; peer dyads	Individual; group
D	Individual; peer group	Individual; peer group	Individual; peer group	Individual; peer group	Individual; peer group
E	Individual; group	Individual	Individual; group	Individual	Individual; group
F	Individual; peer dyads	Group; peer dyads	Individual; peer dyads	Group; peer dyads	Individual; peer dyads
G	Individual	Group	Individual	Group	Individual

cases or has a brief time period for applied practice as in some training programs. In such situations each supervisee can learn from the therapeutic work of others in the supervision group. Furthermore, the availability of support from others is high in group supervision especially because the others are peers and so are experiencing similar difficulties and successes.

Group supervision is also helpful when supervisees are conducting groups of their own and can use the supervision group as a laboratory in which new techniques are tried. Group supervision could be used on a weekly basis to supplement individual supervision as shown in pattern E of Table 1 or on an alternating basis with group supervision one week and individual supervision the next week as shown in pattern G of Table 1.

Peer supervision, whether it is a group or dyad, is another modality that supervisors might use to supplement individual supervision as shown in pattern D of Table 1. The choice of using a group or dyads in peer supervision depends on whether the standard form of group supervision (led by a supervisor) is used. If standard group supervision is already in use then adding peer group supervision is redundant. Peer group supervision is a reasonable alternative to group supervision providing the supervisees are competent group participants and can assume the supervisor or supervisee roles appropriately to help the group attain their goals.

In several community agencies in Philadelphia research has been conducted to observe the effects of peer group supervision among mental health workers (Lear & Hart, 1980). Most of the participants are not skilled group members and have not received clinical supervision in their training or work experience. In order to establish an effective supervisory group they are first learning effective group skills and developing norms such as support and cohesiveness.

If group supervision of the standard format is to be used, then peer supervision should be implemented in dyads as shown in pattern C of Table 1. Dyads could supplement either the standard group supervision or peer group supervision. Peer supervision in dyads allows more individual attention to each peer than is the case in a group. Peer supervision in dyads could also be the sole supplement to individual supervision with the main advantage being that in a peer dyad, supervisees feel less threat of evaluation than with a supervisor.

Peer supervision in a group or dyads can be used on an alternating basis with individual supervision and standard group supervision. For example, individual supervision could take place weekly while group supervision and peer supervision dyads meet every other week in an alternating fashion as shown in pattern C of Table 1. A second example would be to have peer supervision dyads meet weekly and have individual and standard group supervision meet during alternate weeks as shown in pattern F. These decisions must rest with the supervisor's analysis of the supervisees and the goals inherent within the context.

Combinations of Modality and Model

The modality (individual, group, or peer supervision) interacts with the model (Skill Development, Personal Growth, or Integration) making it necessary that supervisors be aware of the effects of various modality-model combinations when choosing a modality. The general goals for supervisees should be established first. Each supervisor then assesses the characteristics of the supervisee, context, and supervisor to select an appropriate model and an appropriate modality. The difficulty lies in choosing the model and modality whose combined effects are more appropriate for a particular group of supervisees than other combinations of model and modality.

The traditional combination of model and modality, especially at the beginning of the supervision process, is to use the Skill Development model with individual supervision as the modality. Many supervisors and supervisees seem to be satisfied with this combination and so have often extended the skill development goals to the group and peer modalities. The basis of this plan is to attain skill development goals via different approaches assuming that each modality will be distinctly different from other modalities and that each modality will promote learning that would not be promoted by the other modalities. Whether this assumption is valid remains to be tested empirically. Another combination of modality and model based on this same assumption, however, is to use the individual, group, and peer modalities to accomplish the goals of either Personal Growth or of Integration.

A different way of combining modalities and models uses several models, each paired with a different modality. For example, the Skill Development model might be used in individual supervision and the Personal Growth model used in group supervision or perhaps peer supervision in a group. A further possibility would be to add the Integration model with peer supervision in dyads. The fundamental concept of this complex pattern is that several goals are important for supervisees to attain. Each of these goals is best accomplished by a separate modality because of the unique characteristic of each modality. Because individual supervision can provide focused attention, skill development can be achieved quite effectively. Groups have a good record of achieving personal growth and so a standard group or a peer supervision group can be used to attain the goals of the Personal Growth model. If supervisors recognize and value the goals of the Integration model, they can be accomplished by means of a standard group, peer group, or peer dyad.

Furthermore, a different modality could be the means of carrying out each of several goals of a particular model. For example, individual supervision could be used to attain the goal of skill acquisition in the Skill Development model while group supervision could be used to accomplish the goal of case conceptualization, which is also a goal within the Skill Development model. Again, the validity of these patterns remains to be tested in terms of how efficiently supervisees learn. Of particular interest is that this latter combination ignores the developmental or evolutionary process of supervision, that is, having supervisees work on several or all goals at once instead of moving from one goal to another in succession. This pattern may work with both skill development and personal growth goals but adding the integration goal seems questionable.

One additional combination of modality and model takes into account the developmental process of supervision. Assuming that most supervisees begin with an expectation of and a request for skill development and then move to an interest in personal growth followed by a concern for integration, supervisors could use different combinations of modalities and models throughout the overall supervision process. For example, a supervisor initially might use the Skill Development model via the individual and/or group and/or peer modalities but then change the model as supervisees are ready to work on personal growth. At this point the supervisor would shift the model in one or all modalities from Skill Development to Personal Growth. Later, the supervisor could change from the Personal Growth to the Integration model in one or more modalities when the supervisees were ready to work on the goal of integration. This flexibility allows for multiple goals to be achieved through several modalities and recognizes the occurrence of developmental stages more than any other combination of modality and model.

In general supervisors should try different combinations of models and modalities to see which ones are appropriate. Future research should compare the processes of these combinations of modality and model as well as the differences in outcomes of these various combinations.

TEMPORAL APPLICATION

Temporal application of a model and modality refers to the timing of supervision in relation to the time therapy sessions are conducted by supervisees. Supervision (modality and model) could be applied in a live (during a therapy session), immediate (immediately following a therapy session), or delayed (a few hours to a week following a therapy session) format. Which of these temporal applications is chosen depends on obvious environmental constraints of the training program or agency and more subtle characteristics of the philosophy of the supervisor about training. Constraints of the training program or agency include lack of space to conduct groups, or lack of observation rooms or videotape equipment, which severely limits the effectiveness of live and immediate supervision. Another constraint might be a schedule of courses and/or clients that restricts people from gathering together to observe each other as in immediate supervision. Supervisors who are aware of the strengths and weaknesses of these three temporal applications, as described in this section, may be motivated to overcome such barriers formed by their agency or program.

A factor more subtle than environmental constraints is the philosophy of the supervisor about the appropriate pedagogy for training mental health workers. The major contribution to one's philosophy of training and supervision is one's philosophy of conducting therapy. For the most part therapists see clients on a once-per-week basis, more frequently in times of a crisis. Consequently, supervisors, who are also therapists by training and experience, tend to adopt the once-per-week supervision session with the delayed format. The effectiveness of this approach seems rarely questioned nor are other approaches considered. If supervisors were to consider the effects of other forms of temporal application, they might begin to experiment with these forms.

The delayed format is appropriate in many cases and can be used as a basis to which other forms are added. Delayed supervision allows for the supervisee to calm any extreme feelings experienced during a therapy session, to reflect on the session, and to plan for the upcoming supervision sessions. If a tape was made of the therapy session, the supervisee (and also the supervisor) may listen to the tape in order to formulate questions and topics to be discussed in supervision. The delayed supervision format also allows for other techniques such as a psychological report, case notes, or a log to be completed in the time between the therapy session and the supervision session.

The immediate application of supervision following a therapy session has certain strengths, yet it should be made clear that immediate supervision would probably take place after one therapy session per week, not after every therapy session a supervisee conducts each week. Assuming that a supervisee conducts several therapy sessions per week, the supervisor and supervisee must choose the appropriate case on which to apply immediate supervision. The cases not selected for immediate supervision should receive attention by some other means such as delayed supervision; unfortunately, this does not always happen.

Immediate supervision, especially when combined with the technique of observation, allows the supervisor to observe the supervisee's therapeutic techniques, the client's dynamics, or emotional expression of the supervisee in a more vivid way than in delayed supervision. The supervisee in immediate supervision is more clearly aware of the events of the therapy session, which is helpful if the Skill Development or Integration models are used. The supervisee is also aware of intense feelings that were stimulated during the therapy session, which is helpful if the Personal Growth or Integration model has been adopted.

The live supervision form of temporal application, like immediate supervision, is probably used with only one of the supervisee's weekly therapy sessions. In live supervision a supervisor, sometimes aided by a group of the supervisee's peers, provides comments and direction to a supervisee during the actual therapy session. In this way the supervisor's comments are closest to the actual therapeutic techniques and feelings of the supervisee displayed with a client. Because of this proximity supervisees are more likely to grasp the meaning of the supervisor's statements. Furthermore, the supervisees can see the effects of their new behavior immediately in the therapy session thus strengthening the likelihood that such new behavior will be maintained in future sessions and generalize to sessions with other clients. Live supervision is especially helpful in attaining the goals of the Skill Development model and the Integration model.

Faced with these three choices of temporal application, a supervisor must decide which combination of model and modality is best suited for each temporal application. It seems that the combination of individual supervision and the Skill Development model (particularly the skill acquisition, not the case conceptualization goal) would be delivered most effectively through live supervision, to a lesser extent through immediate supervision, and to the least extent through delayed supervision. The justification for this speculation is that supervisees can learn and practice skills most effectively when their work with clients is freshest to them. In immediate supervision the details of the therapy session are vivid and in live supervision the supervisee can try out skills suggested by the supervisor. Individual supervision and the Personal Growth model may be most successful when applied in a delayed format and perhaps less successful in the immediate fashion and least successful in the live format. This statement is based on the premise that personal growth requires some distance from the case itself and some time for thoughtful consideration of the supervisee's broader interpersonal functioning with persons other than clients.

The combination of individual supervision and the Integration model probably accomplishes most when applied through the delayed format, less when applied via immediate delayed supervision, and least when applied by means of live supervision. This sequence, like that suggested for the Personal Growth model, is based on the idea that supervisees need to step back from their clients and examine the relationship of personal patterns and professional development in a relaxed and introspective manner. Of course, these speculations are based on observational data and need to be tested in field studies that assess the effectiveness of various temporal applications. The combinations of model, modality, and temporal application can become even more complex than described here, thus complicating the supervisor's decision-making process. Judicious choices of combinations, however, can provide effective means of promoting supervisee development.

One pattern is to use group supervision as a consistent basis by which the Skill Development model is applied through the live supervision format. In essence the strengths of each modality, model, and temporal application are joined. An option is for supervisors to add to this basic pattern individual or peer group supervision to implement the Personal Growth model on a delayed basis, which was the implied suggestion of Gaoni and Neumann (1974). An alternative is to establish a standard group that carries out the Integration model through immediate supervision. This pattern with various options is based on the concept that the supervisor can apply one combination of modality and model through live supervision and a different combination of modality and model through a second form of temporal application. This concept allows for the supervisor to meet multiple goals. A modification of this pattern is based on the idea that for different goals within the same model of supervision learning could be attained more effectively through different temporal applications. For example, skill acquisition, a goal of the Skill Development model, may be achieved with greatest success through live supervision but case conceptualization may be accomplished more successfully through delayed supervision.

Another major pattern uses the developmental process as the underlying foundation for selection of modality, model, and temporal application. The supervisor would begin with the Skill Development model as implemented, for example, by the live supervision format and by standard group or peer group supervision through the immediate or delayed format. Later in the supervisory process, when the supervisees are ready for personal growth experiences the supervisor can apply the Personal Growth model through individual supervision on a delayed basis and through a standard group or a peer group with the delayed format. Still later, the supervisor can implement the Integration model through individual supervision on an immediate basis and through peer dyads, a peer group or a standard group with the immediate format. The ongoing modification of modality and temporal application may be the most creative effort applied to the field of supervision.

CONFLICTS IN SUPERVISION

Some form of conflict between a supervisor, and a supervisee, or among others in the context such as administrators or peers is inevitable. Supervision is an intense experience in which the supervisor, supervisee, and others have certain expectations about appropriate activities and anxiety about the process itself. Expectations about appropriate activities refers to the ideas each person has of what activities in supervision would be beneficial. Beginning supervisees typically expect skill acquisition activities, and supervisors of advanced clinicians commonly expect to work on integration goals. When expectations of various persons are reasonably similar, supervision may proceed smoothly, whereas differences in expectations result in conflict. Discussions of anxiety during supervision are typically focused only on the supervisee, although in fact anxiety may be experienced by supervisors and others in the context. Conflicts stemming from these sources of anxiety are discussed separately here; however, it should be noted that the actual conflicts are inextricably interwoven.

Stemming from the Supervisee

Supervisee anxiety may be thought of as caused by either a belief about the consequences of a certain behavior ("If I make a mistake

I'll be criticized") or by unanticipated insession events. Although anxiety is an inevitable part of all human interactions and typically is not debilitating, anxiety in supervision should be noted by the supervisor as one of the many factors that affects the interaction.

At the Beginning Although expectations and anxiety are interwoven into a complex pattern, examining them separately here may assist supervisors to gain a richer understanding of the origins of conflict from which to develop effective methods of resolving conflict. Expectations and anxiety are particularly difficult issues when they are not clearly identified. For example, some supervisors have not identified their own expectations of supervisees and so cannot convey a clear set of expectations to their supervisees. Often supervisors and supervisees feel anxious during supervision without knowing a reason for this feeling. An initial step at the outset of each supervisory relationship is for the supervisor and supervisee to identify their expectations as clearly as possible. Any differences can then be discussed and an effective compromise can be negotiated.

A further difficulty with expectations is that a supervisee's request for certain activities in supervision may be tied to anxiety about supervision. For example, a supervisee may request didactic feedback out of fear of discussing personal feelings rather than an actual desire for skill acquisition. Supervision based on such fear will have limited effectiveness. In general a supervisor must discuss extensively the supervisee's expectations and requests so that defensiveness can be detected at the beginning of supervision. An effective supervisor will be able to reduce the supervisee's anxiety and to negotiate appropriate goals.

Just as conflict in supervision, in varying degrees, is inevitable, so too is a negotiation process between the parties in conflict. In every supervision session supervisor and supervisee constantly and subtly negotiate about what is discussed and how much each person directs the discussion. Most of this negotiation process, however, is covert and not defined openly by either supervisor or supervisee as a negotiation. Haley (1963) described this covert interaction as a constant characteristic of all interpersonal interactions. Kadushin (1968), with tongue only somewhat in cheek, described this negotiation process as games supervisors and supervisees play. The pay-off in these games is control of the content and/or process of the supervision sessions and the accompanying feelings of power that occur when control is achieved. Through negotiation, although often a subtle process, supervisor and supervisee express their beliefs, expectations, and anticipated goals, and if successful reach an acceptable compromise and a relationship characterized by increased trust and respect. A general recommendation is to make the covert process more overt through openly discussing the opinions of both supervisor and supervisee about the supervision process.

The negotiation process occurs initially over the choice of a goal for supervision, thus affecting the model of supervision adopted. An effective strategy of negotiation that may prevent conflict is for the supervisor and supervisee to form a team that will explore motivations and preferences of the supervisor, supervisee, and context for a particular goal of supervision. The supervisor and supervisee should discuss their prior experiences with supervision, their theoretical orientation to therapy, goals for supervision, and anxiety (if any) about any aspect of supervision. The supervisor should describe the various goals of supervision, explaining that all goals should be accomplished and that working on a certain goal initially does not exclude other goals, but instead postpones them until the initial goal is completed.

Although some initial conflicts can be eliminated by discussing the topics suggested here, other conflicts will occur later in the supervisory process. However, the supervisory relationship in which differences in expectations and anxiety are resolved through open negotiation may proceed with fewer conflicts than a relationship in which conflicts have not been resolved. One example is the issue of evaluation. If the supervisor and supervisee have not reached a resolution of their differences yielding clear procedures for evaluating the supervisee's performance, then the issue of evaluation will resurface at various points in the supervisory process as a source of conflict. The affective side of the evaluation issue must also be attended to so that supervisees trust that the supervisor will not be harsh, petty, or capricious in evaluating the supervisee's performance. If the supervisee's fears are not replaced by trust then evaluation as an issue will reappear regardless of the clarity of the evaluation procedures initially established.

Later in the Process   The resolution of a conflict at the outset of supervision does not guarantee that other conflicts will not appear later in the process; yet, each successful resolution encourages a supervisor and supervisee to resolve subsequent conflicts rather than ignore them. An important corollary to this point is that initial resolution of a conflict does not guarantee that the resolved issue will not reappear later in supervision. For example, supervisees are concerned initially about evaluation and are helped sometimes to resolve this issue. Yet, weeks later supervisees will again raise this issue as if the prior resolution had not occurred. Apparently, resolution of an issue in supervision must be conceptualized as a temporary phenomenon that lasts until the occurrence of a new anxiety that reopens the issue. This conceptualization is in agreement with the evolutionary nature of supervision developed earlier in this text in which issues, like discrete events in supervision such as tape analysis, have different levels of importance as supervision progresses. The reopening of an issue thought to be resolved previously is not indicative of the *same* conflict that appeared at the outset of supervision and was resolved. At this later point some event or series of events has increased the anxiety present within the supervisor and/or supervisee so that it is manifested in one or more ways—one of which is the reopening of a previously resolved issue. Stated as a principle (yet to be tested empirically), issues will stay resolved in supervision to the extent that supervisor and supervisee anxiety remains low or becomes directed to new issues.

Conflicts that arise later in supervision over new issues are countless, but several of the typical conflicts are described here as illustrations along with suggestions for their resolution. One conflict occurs when the supervisor uses a technique that seems to be inconsistent with the agreed-upon model of supervision causing the supervisee to become anxious. By reviewing the goals and subgoals the supervisor can clarify the direction of supervision. By explaining or reviewing the purpose of the supervisory techniques that have been used and are presently in use, the supervisor can help the supervisee understand the supervisor's logic in selecting these techniques. Consequently, the supervisee can move ahead in the supervision process.

Supervisors using the Personal Growth or Integration model are particularly prone to being challenged by supervisees who become distressed when the relationship between personal competence and professional competence is unclear. Although experienced supervisors may agree with Gurk and Wicas (1979), who believe that a "rigid boundary between the personal and professional lives of trainees seems simplistic and artificial (p. 404)" beginning therapists may find such a boundary comforting. Supervisors must also remember that supervisees who initially understand the supervisory model may become anxious when a particular supervisory technique is too threatening. In this case the supervisor needs to suspend the use of this technique until the supervisee is ready to profit by its use. To continue with a technique that is too anxiety-provoking can only increase conflict and weaken the supervisory relationship.

Another situation that promotes conflict in supervision is that supervisees become anxious about their relationship with their supervisor. In some cases this anxiety is expressed through concern about the validity of the supervisory model or techniques being implemented, by resistance to self-disclose personal thoughts or feelings, or by not revealing any information about knowledge or skills that could be criticized by the supervisor. This situation is indicative, for example, of a relationship in which the supervisor's expertise and, perhaps, attitude have created a hierarchy that has become dysfunctional for supervision. For some supervisees a large hierarchical distance means that the supervisor eventually will disperse harsh criticism, which is certainly to be avoided. Of course, it's a rare person who enjoys criticism, but when the hierarchy is too pronounced, some supervisees not only fear the criticism but also fear that they can never be as competent as the supervisor and so become discouraged, frustrated, and withdrawn.

The desire of supervisees to be as competent as they perceive their supervisors to be is a common occurrence. Aspirations of this type are a positive motivation for supervisees to learn the knowledge and skills of their profession; however, supervisees need periodic reinforcement during the learning process or their motivation will fade. When supervisees perceive that their supervisor far outdistances them in professional or personal development, they may retreat and become in conflict with the supervisor.

Supervisors must deemphasize and reduce the hierarchy between themselves and supervisees who have perceived a great distance between them. By disclosing their own therapeutic errors, doubts, and disappointments, supervisors can change supervisees' perceptions of the supervisor from all-competent and all-powerful to reasonably competent and powerful. This revised perception of the supervisor's competence level becomes more attainable for the supervisees. Furthermore, criticism offered by the reasonably competent and powerful supervisor can be accepted and used more effectively than the immobilizing criticism emanating from the all-competent and all-powerful supervisor.

For other supervisees and supervisors, the hierarchy between them will be dysfunctional because the distance is too low. The supervisees may perceive that their supervisor is relatively incompetent as a therapist or relatively low in personal development or integration of the professional and personal realms. In this situation supervisees feel disappointed in the feedback from supervisors because of low credibility they attach to it. Consequently, a conflict develops in which the supervisee becomes resistant to suggestions and supervisory techniques. The supervisor must emphasize and increase the hierarchy in this instance, perhaps by playing a tape, generating a creative hypothesis about a client, role-playing the part of a therapist, or sharing a therapeutic success so that the supervisee will perceive the supervisor as more competent and higher in personal development.

Conflict is also prompted when the supervisee is ready to move to another goal and the supervisor is not. Consequently, the supervisee does less work, is resistant, or expresses the conflict in some other form. For example, a supervisee who has worked on skill development may perceive that at least minimal competence has been attained in this area and wishes to explore the personal area. The supervisor may perceive that the supervisee needs more work on skill development before engaging in personal development, and thus a conflict is formed. Of course, the converse may occur in which the supervisor wants to move to a different goal and the supervisee does not. For example, the supervisor may perceive that the supervisee is ready to engage in integration but the supervisee consistently retreats to skill development or personal growth topics.

In either of the examples given above, the supervisor and supervisee can discuss the conflict, and if their differences are attributable to their disagreement on goals, certain compromises can be established. The supervisor could agree to stay with the supervisee's goal for a certain period of time or until certain skills are attained and then move to the next goal. Or the supervisee could agree to move to the next goal immediately with the option of returning to the prior goal at a later point in time. Changing goals, although common and necessary, is a process sometimes causing conflict that needs resolution.

One final type of conflict arises particularly when the Integration model is being applied. This conflict is attributable to the resistance of supervisees to perceiving that their personal attitudes and feelings affect their clinical behavior. A supervisee may be unaware, for example, of defensive reactions to interpersonal exchanges that occur with clients and others as well. Even after the supervisor has pointed out the supervisee's behavior using videotape playback, the supervisee still may not clearly perceive the behavior as defensive. Another strategy is to use the concept of parallel process to identify the supervisee's behavior as it occurs during the supervision session. For example, Ms. Kelley saw her supervisee, Mr. Jacobson, interrupting silences that had occurred with clients rather than allowing the clients to speak when ready.

Ms. Kelley also noticed that when she pauses to think during supervision sessions Mr. Jacobson quickly picks up the conversation. One day when this took place she pointed it out to Mr. Jacobson and told him that the behavior also takes place with clients. Many supervisees have perceptual blocks toward their own behavior when it is upsetting, and conflict may result when a supervisor uses traditional methods of feedback to identify the supervisee's behavior. Parallel process as a feedback technique is a powerful method of resolving conflict as well as an effective learning strategy even when conflict is not present.

A major concept is that the developmental stage of supervision affects the types of conflicts that occur. In the beginning of supervision both supervisor and supervisee are likely to have conflict over such issues as roles each one is to take, evaluation, goals, and the control each person is to have over the direction taken and content discussed. Later in the process, the conflicts typically arise over feedback given (or not given) to the supervisee, whether goals and subgoals have been achieved, the degree of hierarchy, or new techniques that are anxiety-producing. Much later in supervision when termination is near, conflicts may be present because of reluctance to terminate by the supervisor or supervisee or because of unfulfilled agreements regarding areas to be covered.

In some conflicts the supervisor and supervisee may need the help of an outside consultant who understands supervision and can help clarify the forces producing the conflict and assist the supervisee and supervisor to resolve the conflict. Usually the consultant is used on an as-needed basis to review tapes of the supervision sessions and, perhaps, some tapes of the supervisee's therapy sessions with clients. The consultant would then meet with the supervisor or both supervisor and supervisee to give feedback and clarify the nature of the conflict. Once the supervisor and supervisee understand the conflict, it is assumed that they can resolve it satisfactorily. One use of a consultant, triadic supervision, was described earlier and is more fully described by Spice and Spice (1976) and demonstrated on videotape by Heckel et al. (1975).

Stemming from the Supervisor

Up to this point suggestions for conflict resolution have relied on the supervisor's ability to communicate information to the supervisee that will alter, in some way, the supervisee's perception of supervision (including the supervisor) and thus reduce anxiety. It is important to keep in mind that the simple act of identifying the existence of a conflict is helpful, as is listening to the supervisee's perceptions and feelings in an understanding and caring fashion. These acts help to make known the unknown and also to strengthen a relationship so that other steps toward conflict resolution can take place.

Although the discussion of conflict in supervision has focused, up to this point, on the supervisee, there are also sources of conflict that are precipitated by anxiety within the supervisor and other people in the context in which supervision occurs. The literature in supervision contains virtually no examples of supervisor-initiated conflict although every supervisor has heard complaints about colleagues that seem quite plausible. A few of the typical supervision issues that can create conflict are described here along with some guidelines for avoiding and resolving them.

One of the most prevalent conflicts arises when a supervisor feels frustrated or disappointed by a supervisee's slow progress. Learning to be a competent clinician is a demanding process that proceeds in a halting fashion. Supervisors who expect steady progress by supervisees will find that their expectations will not be realized. The conflict is not the fault of the supervisee, who would probably enjoy a smooth growth process, but that of the supervisor whose ideals have not been met. The conflict must be brought to the surface and discussed so that the supervisor can revise those expectations to include periodic errors and setbacks by the supervisee. It would even be wise for the supervisor to tell the supervisee that progress will be slow at times and that setbacks will occur so that the supervisee can cope with these events more effectively when they take place.

Another kind of conflict occurs when the supervisor becomes competent at working with a particular set of skills or with a certain client population or with a specific level of supervisee training and now must adjust to a new group. For example, a supervisor might have become quite competent and comfortable supervising beginning clinicians in basic skills, but to switch to a more advanced group wanting higher order skills could be distressing, thus resulting in conflict with specific supervisees. Similarly, a supervisor could be well-versed in the use of diagnostic techniques with children but when called upon to supervise a person wanting to learn family therapy skills, the supervisor might well experience some insecurity and anxiety. One recommendation for supervisors faced with this situation, as in other situations they encounter, is to be honest with the supervisee about areas of expertise. The next step is to make the learning of the needed skills a joint venture between supervisor and supervisee so that the supervisor does not have to feign knowledge or competence and thus perpetuate an unspoken conflict. Because the supervisor has a basic repertoire of supervisory skills, these skills can be applied to a new group of clients or set of clinical skills if the supervisor is willing to learn along with the supervisee.

The idea that supervisors can be effective even though the supervisor is not an expert at the particular task, or has not worked with a specific client problem or has not resolved the particular personal issue faced by the supervisee, is in sharp contrast to the long-accepted notion that a clinician cannot help others until first having gained the necessary skill, insight, or integration. The main aim of supervision as an enabling process, however, is not to teach skills per se or resolve personal conflicts; rather, supervision assists clinicians to evaluate their personal and professional behavior so that they can themselves seek out new meaning and alternatives in their interactions. Although much of what is termed *supervision* is in reality teaching or therapy, the person conducting supervision as described in this text can assist supervisees in becoming more professionally competent even though he or she has not attained the highest levels of professional development.

Conflict also occurs when the supervisee exceeds or is perceived to exceed the supervisor in level of either skills, personal growth, or integration. Although it is unlikely that a supervisee would be advanced in all areas, supervisees can and will excel in certain skills or conceptualizations, in their personal insight or affective sensitivity, or in their integration of their professional and personal characteristics. When a supervisee's level of competence exceeds that of the supervisor, a conflict could result. Some supervisors may recognize the difference in competence with feelings of pride coupled with envy. Other supervisors may become anxious without recognizing the cause, thereby precipitating a conflict. Often, the anxious supervisor stops rewarding the supervisee or even raises the standards for success, thus frustrating and disappointing the supervisee. Of the conflicts initiated by the supervisor described so far, this conflict is one of the most difficult for the supervisor to realize and resolve. The conflict may become severe enough so that both supervisor and supervisee agree to seek the help of a consultant, or they may terminate supervision. Some supervisees may try to mask or even denigrate their attainment of competence in order to reduce the supervisor's anxiety and thus the overt conflict. Periodic self-evaluation and peer review by supervisors of their performance can help to prevent a conflict of this nature.

Another way to conceptualize the conflict of the supervisees becoming superior to the supervisor in a particular area is in terms of hierarchy. It is assumed that at the outset of most supervisory relationships the supervisor is superior to the supervisee in level of skill, personal growth, and integration, although this assumption is probably not justified universally. Nevertheless, the supervisor enters the relationship at a hierarchical position above that of the supervisee. For some supervisors this position is quite comfortable and they wish to maintain it; however, when the supervisee surpasses the supervisor in some area, the hierarchy is reduced thus threatening the supervisor's once comfortable position. To reestablish the hierarchical distance, supervisors resort to criticizing the supervisee, raising the standards for success, or embellishing their own level of skill, personal growth, or integration by describing some professional or personal accomplishment.

In the opposite way, other supervisors feel uncomfortable with the usually high level of hierarchical distance established at the outset of supervision and so attempt to reduce and even eliminate the hierarchy by becoming the supervisee's friend. A possible motivation for a supervisor's attempt to diminish the hierarchical distance by establishing a friendship is that the supervisor wishes to prevent the supervisee from becoming (or at least admitting to) more competence than the supervisor. A supervisee might surpass a supervisor but how could a friend surpass another friend? The so-called friendship may be yet another way that conflict is kept on a covert level and so more difficult to identify. Most supervisors wish to have smooth relationships rather than ones filled with conflict and so may keep conflicts from surfacing even though supervisee learning may suffer.

Stemming from the Context

Every conflict between a supervisor and a supervisee exists within a context that, to some degree, supports or does not support the initiation and continuation of that conflict. Because all supervision exists within a context the influence of the context is inevitable. The difficulty in analyzing this influence is that the supervisor and supervisee variables cannot be held constant to allow the differential impact of the context to be noted. Some contexts, however, present certain conditions that initiate conflict in supervisory relationships having no prior conflict or further conflicts in supervisory relationships in which conflict already is present. Several of these conditions are examined here to illustrate the types of context factors that promote conflict between supervisors and supervisees.

The most important factor in the context affecting supervisor-supervisee conflict is the resistance of the context to change. It is assumed that every group, whether in a training program or comminity agency, has a homeostatic balance that the majority of the group wishes to maintain. Consequently, change of any sort is viewed as threatening to the balance and so is resisted. Haley (1975) and Liddle (1978) describe in clear detail their efforts to initiate change within organizations and the resistance that they encountered. Of course, efforts to change occur in a variety of forms but several forms seem particularly involved with supervision.

One form of change to which contexts react strongly is innovations in either the model, techniques, modality, or temporal application of supervision. For example, one faculty member conducted a demonstration to the faculty of how videotape could be used to record role-play sessions in a practicum and then provide feedback to the supervisees on their clinical skills. At the end of the demonstration a senior faculty member proceeded to describe how difficult and time-consuming the tape recording process was. The faculty member then moved into the artificiality of the taping and finally closed with the statement that sensitive and perceptive supervisors could provide the same feedback without all the bother of using equipment. The message of resistance, regardless of the validity of the counterarguments, was clear. (The group did evolve over the next few years to use audiotape and videotape recording for training and supervision but not with complete agreement among all group members.)

Supervisors who use innovative techniques, such as videotape in the example above, identify themselves as different from other supervisors. Although a supervisor did not set out initially to acquire this label, the label is attached. Those supervisors who are different experience pressure from the rest of the group, and these pressures manifest themselves in the relationship between supervisor and supervisee. For example, the innovative supervisor may show feelings of cautious optimism or rebellious anger with supervisees in response to the pressures of the context. Supervisees are likely to react negatively when faced by these feelings. Similarly, supervisees may perceive that their supervisor is "different" in a pejorative sense rather than "innovative," which has a more positive connotation. Their feelings could range from embarrassment to fear of being supervised in a way that is so different from that of their peers.

Conflict may also be noted between the non-innovative supervisors and their supervisees. One doctoral student completed her didactic and experiential work on campus and went to her year-long internship in a community agency. During the first meeting with her supervisor she described her previous clinical work in which she found live supervision and videotape feedback to be of particular value in her development of skills. The new supervisor seemed distressed and then admitted that he had no knowledge of or training in these supervisory methods. In this case a potential conflict was avoided by the supervisor's openness; other supervisors may not have been so quick to admit their deficits. These supervisors may well experience distress that later precipitates a conflict as supervisees ask "Why don't we try some of these supervisory methods?"

One adjunctive point regarding successful supervisors in a particular context is that any successful supervisor will be resented or envied by some coworkers. Depending on the number in the group with these feelings and the intensity of the feelings, pressure will be directed, albeit subtly in most cases, toward the successful supervisor to either stop being successful or else to make the successes less noticeable. This pressure could then be manifested in the supervisor's relationship with supervisees.

A different but also powerful condition in contexts that precipitates and heightens conflict between supervisor and supervisee is the difference between the goal of organizational efficiency and the goal of organizational effectiveness. Organizational efficiency of either training program or agency means the maximum use of all available resources to accomplish the tasks of the organization with minimum difficulty. Because efficiency is ultimately tied to financial resources, each organization must determine the quality of service it wishes to deliver for its available finances. When financial resources decline or costs rise, the organization must decide to what degree it will increase revenues and/or decrease costs. Because most agencies and training programs find it difficult to increase revenues, they typically turn to reducing costs. Although reducing costs by improving the efficiency of the organization does not necessarily reduce the extent and/or quality of the services provided, too often "efficiency" is defined in a way that has this effect. In some contexts efficiency is shown by large supervisee-to-supervisor ratios, large client loads, low salaries, and little space and/or equipment for supervision.

Organizations that work to become more efficient by, for example, increasing the number of supervisees per supervisor from 3 to 4 (or from 19 to 20) may not decrease drastically the quality of service, but any change can precipitate or further extend existing conflict between the supervisor and supervisee. The balance between organizational efficiency and organizational effectiveness is difficult to maintain, and the decline of organizational effectiveness can lower morale and promote conflict that inevitably surfaces between supervisor and supervisee.

In all cases of conflict between supervisor and supervisee, conflict can be effectively reduced by supervisors who have been trained to expect conflict and then to reduce conflict. This conflict resolution process should be a component of every comprehensive training experience for supervisors and supervisors-to-be.

TRAINING THE SUPERVISOR

One impetus for the study of supervision has been from the supervisor in the field who wants to be more competent and from the agency director who asks for qualified supervisors to fill positions. Whatever motivations exist, the point is clear that longevity of service or therapeutic expertise is not enough to qualify for a position as a supervisor nor to fulfill effectively the duties of that position as required by the agency director and the supervisees. The Peter Principle, however, applies to the mental health field as well as to business (Peter & Hull, 1969). Consequently, clinicians are often appointed to supervisory positions even though they lack competence in the duties demanded of that position. Of course, one of the prerequisites to any training program in supervision should be a solid understanding by the clinician of his or her theoretical framework used in clinical work. All too often this theoretical understanding is nonexistent. Training programs at universities and in community agencies need to ensure that competent supervisors are also competent clinicians.

A further source of input regarding effective training for supervisors is professional organizations such as the American Psychological Association, American Personnel and Guidance Association, American Psychiatric Association, and National Association of Social Workers. These organizations profess to enhance the professional mental health worker's skills and knowledge and so can be an effective force in establishing guidelines for the training of supervisors and criteria on which to assess the competence of practicing supervisors throughout their careers. Organizations of particular importance are the Association for Counselor Education and Supervision and the American Association for Marriage and Family Therapy.

The Association for Counselor Education and Supervision, a division of the American Personnel and Guidance Association, is composed largely of university faculty members, who train school and agency counselors at the masters degree level, counseling psychologists at the doctoral level, and supervisors in schools and agencies. The journal of this organization, *Counselor Education and Supervision* contains research and innovative practices that are based on the field of psychology. No other field has a journal completely devoted to training and supervision. The Association for Counselor Education and Supervision has also been active in promoting cooperation among professional organizations regarding continuing education for educators and supervisors (Hart, 1978a, 1979b).

The American Association for Marriage and Family Therapy is composed of university faculty, therapists in agencies, and supervisors with backgrounds in social work, pastoral counseling, psychology, or psychiatry. A special category of membership—Approved Supervisor—has been established that is based on training and experience as a supervisor of marriage and family therapists in addition to the regular requirements for clinical membership. This special category is an important step in promoting the belief that didactic and experiential training in supervision beyond therapeutic competence is necessary for effective supervisors.

Professional organizations usually adopt standards for competence that are based on the recommendation of leading university faculty members and recognized experts from community agencies. Standards usually include references to knowledge of theory and hours of supervised practice. Unfortunately, universities and agencies do not frequently consult each other regarding the implementation of standards; therefore, university goals are criticized as unrealistic, and agency goals are criticized as lacking innovation. A cooperative effort is needed so that goals and specific supervisory competencies can be created; then, the implementation of these goals and competencies can be addressed. Effective supervision in the future will be determined, in part, by the extent of cooperation in goal formation by universities and agencies.

Goals

It is apparent that supervisors-in-training should achieve several goals. A list of goals is presented here as an initial step in the formation of a more comprehensive list of goals. Goals for supervisors-in-training would include:

Knowledge of models, modalities, and temporal application of
    supervision

Knowledge of the developmental process of supervision

Knowledge of the characteristics that affect the supervisory process, that is, the supervisor, supervisee, and context in which supervision is conducted

Knowledge of supervisory techniques including the appropriate application of these techniques in terms of sequencing, combining, and evaluating the techniques

Knowledge of one's personal relationship patterns and the thoughts and feelings that arise during interactions with supervisees

Integration of knowledge in the areas described here with one's knowledge of his or her personal relationship style

Knowledge of ethical principles that apply to the practices of supervision

Other goals and subgoals could be added, but this list is meant to serve as a basic outline of what supervisors should know. Specific competencies could be delineated for each goal and subgoal. How these goals are implemented is a separate issue.

Implementation of Goals

A central concept in the formation and implementation of goals is that although goals may remain constant, information to be taught changes as professions acquire knowledge about supervision through research and add innovative practices and techniques. The specific knowledge and skills attained by supervisors trained today must be viewed as temporary. Supervisors must accept the reality that competence is not permanently established at the conclusion of a training program but must be continually renewed through inservice activities of a formal and informal nature (Hart, 1979a).

A first step is for universities to add the goals of clinical supervision to their established clinical program. In this way students learning to be psychologists, for example, would have a fundamental knowledge of supervision that could be supplemented at their place of future employment. Later, as these students move into supervisory positions additional goals may be acquired by means of inservice experiences. It is hoped that agencies, professional organizations, and universities will establish workshops, courses, and other activities that allow advanced supervisory goals to be attained.

The goals of supervision listed here can be attained through numerous forms of didactic and/or experiential instruction. Didactic instruction through formal courses and seminars can be supplemented by independent reading, lectures, and workshops and by participation in research in supervision. Experiential instruction consists of being a supervisee and being a supervisor. Being a supervisee refers to experiencing clinical supervision through as many models, modalities, and temporal applications as possible, whereas being a supervisor refers to practicing supervisory skills in simulated and actual situations. Experiential instruction is of particular importance and should be implemented according to the following guidelines.

The first principle regarding experiential instruction in clinical supervision is that having been a supervisee is not the sole criterion for becoming a supervisor although it is a necessary factor. A supervisee acquires a certain knowledge and awareness about the process of supervision that can be acquired only by being a supervisee. Thus, experience as a supervisee should be mandatory. Furthermore, this experience should include contact with as many models, modalities, temporal applications, and techniques as possible. A diversity of experience as a supervisee should promote a wider range of behavior as a supervisor.

Another principle is that training in supervision should start with simulated activities designed to achieve acquisition of supervisory skills and later move to the more complicated reality of actual supervision. Simulated activities would include case studies and taped supervisee statements (Hart, 1974; Fitch, Malley, & Scott, 1975; Hart, 1976d, 1976e; Hart et al., 1976d, 1976e) to which supervisors respond orally or in writing. More advanced activities would include role-playing. After sufficient success has been attained at simulation activities, each student would take responsibility for supervising actual supervisees who are working as clinicians. This sequence from simulated to actual practice allows for students to attain skills gradually and with steadily increasing responsibility that keeps anxiety to a minimum.

A further principle is for students to work with all models, modalities, and temporal applications as suggested by Bernard (1979). Each student should have a minimum of two supervisees for individual supervision. Having two supervisees allows the supervisor to examine the differences between the supervision conducted with each supervisee and to consider different approaches that need to be used in either case. Doctoral students in psychology typically supervise masters degree students who are doing fieldwork in an agency. This procedure works well although the experience is not totally realistic because the student-supervisor rarely has administrative responsibility for the supervisee. The lack of this responsibility, however, has the advantage of allowing the novice supervisor to have one less barrier to overcome in establishing a relationship with the supervisees. Furthermore, each student should also conduct a supervision group with another student as a co-leader. In this way the student can contrast group with individual and peer supervision while enjoying the support from the relationship with a peer. Familiarity with peer supervisory dyads or a group can be gained by assisting other faculty members who have established and are now monitoring a peer group or dyads. In addition each student should be asked to conduct supervision sessions that are live, immediate, and delayed so that the different skills in using these formats may be acquired. In order to work with all these modalities and temporal applications, the earlier principle of beginning with the less complex and moving to the more complex should be followed. Students should begin with individual supervision and later add a supervisory group and then peer dyads or peer groups.

One final principle is that supervision of the supervisors-in-training should employ the various modalities, temporal applications, and techniques available. For example, supervisors could be individually supervised by a faculty member who used live, immediate, or delayed supervision. The faculty member should also conduct group supervision with all of the supervisors-in-training concurrent with individual supervision for each of them. Peer supervision may also be used in addition to or on an alternating basis with group supervision. If supervision is a valuable learning process for clinicians, then it should be valuable for supervisors also.

Even as clinicians assume supervisory responsibilities in a particular community agency, new concepts are established and innovative techniques that supervisors should learn are created in the field. A comprehensive program of inservice training, like that for clinicians described by Hart (1979a), should also be formed for supervisors. Such a program could include ongoing case conferences (Loganbill, 1979), peer group dyads or triads (Delworth, 1979), and standard format group supervision; it could include visits by consultants to teach specific concepts or techniques in supervision, and courses, workshops, or lectures on supervision. Many other methods exist by which inservice training can continually upgrade supervisory knowledge and skills as part of a person's continual professional development.

The goal of increased personal awareness in the training of supervisors is similar to the personal growth goal in the training of clinicians. Disturbing as well as pleasant thoughts and feelings arise among supervisors in their interactions with supervisees;

these need to be explored. Those working with supervisors-in-training should allow ample time for discussion of the supervisor-in-training's thoughts and feelings and actively promote such a discussion.

Similarly, the supervisor-in-training should achieve the goal of integrating supervisory skills and knowledge with personal awareness in an authentic and spontaneous style. The techniques used to accomplish this goal can be the same as those used to promote integration among clinicians-in-training.

The last goal listed as necessary for supervisors to attain is a knowledge of guidelines that apply to the ethical practice of supervision. Although professional organizations have established ethical guidelines for general practice of a profession, until recently no specific guidelines have been established for supervisors. In 1979 the North Atlantic Region of the Association for Counselor Education and Supervision (NARACES) began work on ethical guidelines for supervisors. The Pennsylvania Association for Counselor Education and Supervision Committee on Ethical Guidelines for Supervisors, chaired by Dr. Lewis Morgan, compiled a list of guidelines that was adopted by NARACES at its annual meeting in the fall of 1979. These guidelines have been forwarded to the executive council of the Association for Counselor Education and Supervision for their consideration. The guidelines, in Appendix A, are an important step in assisting supervisors to know the parameters of their work and how to proceed in situations in which ethical principles are in question.

DIRECTIONS FOR FUTURE RESEARCH

Research in supervision presently consists of unrelated fragments that make integration difficult and the establishment of meaningful principles impossible. Supervision research, like research on other topics, has been fragmented by the differences in philosophies of various mental health fields and the rivalry that prevents people from cooperating with those who have different training or beliefs. Fragmentation has also come about through differences in the choice of appropriate topics to be researched, which has led to studies that are so situation-specific as to be nongeneralizable or so general as to have no practical application to any particular group or individual. This section contains a description of some of the problems supervision research faces and some guidelines for how future research should be conducted.

"Nothing's been done on this topic" is a frequently-heard comment by researchers. This statement usually means that the researcher reviewed a journal or two in one specific field and found no articles on the topic in question. Researchers often fail to look outside their own field for information, thus useless duplication and repetition instead of valuable replication abound and the progress of knowledge occurs more slowly than necessary. Researchers in supervision in the separate fields of psychiatry, psychology, and social work have not examined and integrated the research that each group has conducted. No doubt this failure has been attributable, in part, to lack of collegial contact among the professions and lack of time and energy to survey the mountain of information that is available. Several suggestions may improve this situation.

Professional organizations typically assemble a variety of research topics, sometimes including supervision, to be presented at their meetings and in their journals. Unless one attends all the meetings or regularly reads all the journals, many presentations on supervision go unnoticed. It would be helpful to have an abstracting service that would pull out articles, papers presented at national meetings, dissertations, and books that focus on some aspect of supervision. Computer-assisted searches of the literature are useful but are only as good as the number and type of sources they tap.

A further suggestion is to conduct national and regional meetings on supervision that include researchers and practioners from all fields. In this way people could hear diverse points of view and be assured that the conference would be sufficiently narrow in scope as to warrant the time and expense of attending. A related suggestion is to establish a journal on supervision that solicits articles from all fields. Because journals typically serve the interests of a particular professional group, they have a parochial quality that excludes information from other fields. A new journal could operate independently on a subscription basis and would accept a wide range of articles on supervision. All fields of mental health might be willing to participate in the advancement of this topic, if its prominence were increased by the establishment of a central organization for researchers and writers.

One further difficulty in the research on supervision is the variety of philosophies that guide the conduct of research in general. The historical tradition within psychiatry and social work leads to extensive case study and descriptive studies from which principles can be abstracted. These principles, however, are not always immediately useful to supervisors with individual supervisees. On the other hand, research from some psychologists examines highly specific cause and effect relationships so that effective practices can be determined; however, the principles on which these practices are based remain unspecified. Research strategies should seek first to prove or disprove the assumptions on which all practices are based and then evaluate the practices that emerge from the assumptions that hold true.

Definitions

Researchers must first clarify the definitions of concepts that are frequently used throughout the literature in psychiatry, social work, and psychology. One of the biggest issues is that researchers study supervisors who are experienced and thus equate "experience" with "expertise." Many of these supervisors are untrained and may well be less effective than the recent graduate clinician who received specific training in supervision. Assumptions cannot be made about the quality of the supervision or the supervisor based solely on the supervisor's years of service. Indeed, level of experience should be examined (Smith, 1975) as one of the supervisor characteristics that may affect the supervision process but should not be equated with expertise.

Years of supervisory experience should be examined more carefully thus questioning the idea that "more is better." As Gelso (1979) suggested, the effects attributed to the supervisor's experience in actuality may be attributable to the supervisor's age or physical appearance. In contrast, supervisee experience is rarely examined or even noted. Most research is done on beginning supervisees in university training programs, and to generalize these research results to experienced supervisees working in agencies is unjustified. By studying levels of experience of the supervisor and supervisee and their interaction the supervision process as a whole may be clarified.

A further confusion in definitions results from studies of supervision, usually in psychology, that are actually studies of group instruction. In many university training programs, eight to ten (or more) students at the masters degree level meet, usually weekly, for several hours in a practicum seminar. Students typically see clients outside the university in a school or agency field work placement and report on their activities to the seminar. The actual amount of time spent in clinical supervision, as opposed to administrative supervision, assimilation to the mores of the profession, or emotional adjustment to the training program or field work site often is minimal. Generalizations about clinical supervision based on practicum seminars are highly questionable. Researchers must investigate sessions where clinical supervision is the primary task.

Methodological Issues

One of the many issues researchers must consider is the field study versus the laboratory study. Researchers should be careful of moving too quickly into the laboratory to isolate variables and control for the many factors that exist in field studies. The laboratory study often relies on linear or simple cause-and-effect principles derived from the classic animal studies on conditioning. This conceptualization however, portrays human behaviors as discrete (i.e., separate from each other) and as continuous (i.e., repeated with relative sameness across situations). This conceptualization is challenged by the ecosystem idea that behaviors are meshed with each other and cannot be pulled out singly for examination without destroying any meaningful understanding of how these behaviors operate in reality.

Furthermore, the systemic notion suggests that behaviors are constantly changing, albeit subtly and slowly, because of the force of pressures within a person's environment. Change is seen as inevitable, ongoing, and pervasive. Consequently, researchers may find that field studies are much more useful in understanding the range of variables that affects supervisor and supervisee change. Furthermore, researchers may realize that the laboratory study is not completely free from the variables that are present in the field. It is wise to remember Thoresen's warning: "Justification for claiming that a causal relationship has been demonstrated in *any* experiment or series of experiments is very precarious, regardless of design" (Thoresen, 1979, p. 59).

Gelso (1979) supported Bordin's (1974) suggestion that "The degree to which we can safely depart from the naturalistic setting is proportional to the amount we already know about the phenomena in question" (Gelso, 1979, p. 15). Therefore, it is not only appropriate but also essential that careful field study be done before conducting the analogue study in the laboratory. In typical analogue studies researchers examine a supervisor's responses to written case studies, a supervisee on tape, or a coached supervisee. Not only are these studies conducted in an atypical setting but also they often are one-shot events rather than segments of an ongoing process. Thus, the "supervisor" in the study has no historical perspective on the "supervisee" and no need for expectations about the future. Gelso (1979) advocated, instead, the field experiment, in which subjects (clients, supervisees) are randomly assigned to two or more groups and, although the study takes place in a natural setting, the researcher maintains control of the "when and to whom" the independent variable is exposed. In comparison to the experimental analogue, the correlational analogue, and the correlational field study, Gelso (1979) concluded that "this field experiment is *potentially* the most powerful of the four basic research strategies" (p. 16).

In summary, research in supervision must describe in detail the interactive process during supervision as well as the results outside of supervision. Research in supervision has moved too quickly into laboratory based analogue studies where discrete variables are examined in a simple linear fashion. Usually such studies have concluded that "more is better" and that the "more clearly" information and expectations are presented, the more supervisees achieve.

The notion that "more is better" refers to the quantitative fact that more change results when clinicians receive supervision than when they don't. To prove continually that people receiving some form of treatment will change more than people who receive no such treatment seems of little value. A much more intriguing issue is the qualitative one—what is the nature of the various changes and what factors contribute to their occurrence.

The idea of "the clearer the better" means that supervisees who are told what to learn and that their supervisor wants them to learn it achieve greater gains in learning compared with supervisees receiving ambiguous instruction and unclear supervisor expectations. This pedagogical truism has been known in educational psychology for many years and has been validated by research in microcounseling by Ivey (1978). It need not be rediscovered by those conducting supervision research. A more important issue for examination would be how the clarity of the supervisor statements regarding expectations is affected by the expectations of the supervisee and the context.

One of the most important recommendations regarding the conduct of research is to move to the examination of individual supervisor and supervisee verbal interactions as the focus of inquiry. The process of supervision typically has been assessed in terms of the supervisor-supervisee relationship as measured by supervisor and/or supervisee self-reports. A common alternative to self-reports is observer ratings, usually of the supervisor's expression of therapeutic conditions. By assessing the supervisor's and supervisee's statements together as a unit (see the thought unit described by Danish, D'Augelli, & Brock, 1976) and relating the unit to salient concepts such as supervisory model, the supervisory process may be understood in the complex manner in which it exists. Once the immediate supervisor-supervisee interaction process is more clearly understood, the later outcomes of supervision on the supervisee and on clients can be related to the insession interaction process with more confidence.

Gelso (1979) describes eight continua on which criteria for assessing research hypotheses may be placed. The internal-external continuum (perhaps a dichotomy rather than a continuum) refers to internal criteria, which measure the insession behaviors of counselor and client (or supervisor and supervisee) and external criteria, which assess out-of-session behavior by the participants, usually the client. Closely related to this continuum is the immediate-ultimate dimension. Immediate refers to criteria used immediately during the counselor-client interaction as is the case with so-called process research. Mediate criteria are those that are used to assess change that may have occurred over a series of counselor-client interactions. Ultimate criteria, such as ideal states of existence, like self-actualization are the end result of the steps taken by clients in counseling and are measured following the counseling process. These two continua are a helpful way of conceptualizing research in contrast to the often misleading process-outcome dichotomy. Researchers must decide on the particular point at which an outcome is to be assessed (immediate, mediate, or ultimate) and whether the assessment should be made within the supervisory session (internal) or outside the session (external). These decisions are based, of course, on the particular question the study has been designed to answer.

Characteristics of both the supervisor and supervisee affect the interaction that occurs between them. Aspects of the supervisor that should be studied are level of training/skills, level of experience, therapeutic orientation, expectations about supervision (of both supervisor and supervisee), and interpersonal behavior patterns including the expression of facilitative conditions. As suggested earlier, therapeutic orientation of the supervisor should be studied to see how, if at all, this characteristic is related to one's choice of model and to one's behavior toward supervisees when using various models. The first step would be to examine a large number of supervisors having a wide range of theoretical orientations to determine their typical model of supervision. An analysis of this data would reveal whether supervisors with a particular therapeutic orientation chose one model more than others. With a sufficiently large sample a multivariate analysis could be conducted in order to determine how much each factor and combination of factors contributes to the choice of a model.

Aspects of the supervisee to be examined include expectations (of themselves and the supervisor), level of training and experience, patterns of interpersonal behavior, and learning styles. Learning style refers to speed and efficiency with which supervisees can acquire various types of information. Some supervisees are able to learn best from principles that are discussed and demonstrated and others learn best by critiques of their performance with clients. Skillful teachers modify their approaches to reach students with different learning styles, and supervisors should be similarly advised. Learning styles, like other interpersonal patterns, are an important consideration in selecting supervisory techniques. Research investigations should include consideration of learning style as one of the important variables affecting the process of supervision.

The impact of these supervisor and supervisee characteristics must then be compared with the impact of the model used by the supervisor. It may turn out that a certain percent of a supervisee's learning is determined by the relationship with the supervisor, a certain percent by the model of supervision and a certain percent by other aspects. Comparing the effects of various aspects of the supervisor process will help researchers and supervisors consider supervision as a composite of many factors, not just one, and the dangers of oversimplification can be avoided.

Once some general descriptions of supervision have been gained through examinations of supervisor and supervisee self-reports, the next step is to examine insession behavior of supervisors and supervisees. Attempts to predict or describe their behavior from data gathered by traditional assessment techniques (such as pencil-and-paper measures of global personality variables) will have little worth. Self-report measures have little relationship to overt behavior and, therefore, give little help in understanding the supervisor's particular behavioral impact on supervisees. Numerous scales exist such as ones listed by Simon and Boyer (1970). The Hart (1979b) Supervision Assessment Scale is in Appendix B.

Research in supervision typically has used the pretest-posttest design (Campbell & Stanley, 1963). University students, for example, are assessed at the beginning and end of a 10-to-15 week supervision experience. This design detects gross change but does not show the variety of changes that may have occurred throughout the time period. The implicit assumption of researchers using this design is that change occurs in a linear (rather than a curvilinear) fashion—an assumption that needs to be questioned. Research in supervision could be strengthened by using interim assessments throughout the supervisory process in order to examine the process of change more thoroughly.

Furthermore, studies are usually conducted within a relatively brief time period, usually equal to the length of a term within a university calendar. The results of a 3-month supervisory experience, however, may not be a condensed version of a year-long experience, but in fact may be only the beginning part of a longer developmental process. Supervision should be studied in time periods of at least 3 months and also up to 12 months if the developmental process of supervision is to be examined adequately.

A final point is that researchers work for long periods of time with small and infrequent rewards and suffer the disappointments and confusion of mixed results. The struggle to bring supervision research into the spotlight of professional review has brought results only in the past 5 years. It is hoped that supervision will, in the future, receive the full attention it deserves.

SUMMARY

Although research studies in supervision have been difficult to compare and often have been unrelated to accepted behavioral theories, some directions have been charted. Supervisors are advised to consider various aspects of the supervisee, supervisors, and context in order to choose the most appropriate model of supervision. Another choice for the supervisor is that of modality (individual, group, or peer supervision) and the combinations of these modalities. A further choice is the temporal application (live, immediate, or delayed) of the model and modality with respect to the time of the therapy session conducted by a supervisee. In addition, the choice of model, modality, and temporal application must be reconsidered at points throughout the supervisory process. As the process evolves, new and different goals for supervisees are created.

Conflict between supervisor and supervisee inevitably arises over the model, modality, or temporal application. Supervisors should be aware of the many causes of conflict and the variety of ways by which the present conflict can be eliminated and by which future conflicts can be prevented.

If supervisors are to combine models, modalities, and temporal applications effectively, and to resolve conflicts successfully, trial-and-error learning should be replaced by systematic training in supervision. This training should occur via university programs and inservice activities in community agencies. Furthermore, the goals for minimal competence in supervision described in this chapter should be continually maintained by ongoing educational activities. In this way supervisors can keep abreast of new techniques and the current thinking developed by other practioners and researchers.

Research in supervision must clarify the vague definitions that have impeded researchers from learning from each other. Coupled with improved research designs and methodology, researchers can bring supervision as a field of study into a place of prominence demanded by their colleagues in the field.

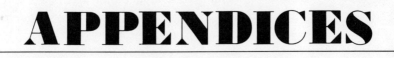

APPENDICES

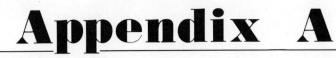

Appendix A

Ethical Standards for Counselor Educators and Supervisors

PREAMBLE

The North Atlantic Association for Counselor Education and Supervision (NARACES) is composed of persons who are engaged in the professional preparation of counselors or who are responsible for supervision of counselors.

Although Ethical Standards have been adopted by the American Personnel and Guidance Association (1974), NARACES recognizes that counselor educators and supervisors carry out responsibilities and activities unique to their job roles and encounter situations which present challenges for implementing ethical standards. These unique situations require the statement of standards especially appropriate for them.

The specification of ethical standards appropriate for Association for Counselor Education and Supervision (ACES) members living in the North Atlantic region enables them to focus on ethical responsibilities held in common, to clarify for present and future members and to those served by members the nature of those ethical standards.

COUNSELING

1. Counselor educators' and supervisors' primary obligation is the training and supervision of trainees and counselors so that they respect the integrity and promote the welfare of the counselees they serve.
2. Counselor educators and supervisors must ensure that their trainees respect the human rights of their counselees, including protecting their rights to privacy and confidentiality in the counseling relationship and information resulting from it.
3. Records of the counseling relationship including interview notes, test data, correspondence, tape recordings, and other documents are to be considered professional information for use in counseling, research, and the training and supervision of counselors, but always with full protection of the identity of the counselee. When it is impossible to protect the identity of the counselee, the written consent of the counselee (or parents, if a minor) must be secured for their use for instructional and research purposes.

RESEARCH

1. Counselor educators and supervisors, in reporting research results, must protect the identity of the subjects.

2. Counselor educators and supervisors shall adhere to current professional and legal guidelines when conducting research with human subjects.
3. In supplying data to aid in the research of another professional, counselor educators and supervisors must observe the ethical and legal rights of the counselee to confidentiality and privacy.
4. Publications by counselor educators and supervisors that include data from other sources shall not only observe fully all copyright laws but shall follow the principle of giving full credit to all to whom credit is due.
5. Counselor educators and supervisors are responsible for conducting and reporting their investigations in a manner that ensures proper interpretation of the data. Explicit mention must be made of all variables and conditions which affect interpretation of the data.
6. Counselor educators and supervisors must honor commitments made to research subjects in return for their cooperation.
7. Training programs should include preparation in research and provide opportunities for the trainee to conduct research that will add to the knowledge in their field.

PERSONNEL ADMINISTRATION

1. Counselor educators and supervisors must pursue professional and personal in-service development through advanced course work, seminars, workshops and professional conferences.
2. Counselor educators and supervisors should regularly submit their own work for review through supervision, peer evaluation, or consultation.
3. Counselor educators and supervisors have an obligation to inform their students and supervisees of the policies, goals, and programs toward which their institutional operations are oriented.
4. Counselor educators and supervisors should require that trainees and supervisees function in a competent manner, compatible with their skills and experiences.
5. Professional competencies expected of trainees shall be communicated in writing prior to admission to the graduate program and to individual courses.
6. Counselor educators and supervisors shall establish training programs which integrate academic study and supervised practice.

7. Counselor educators and supervisors, through continual trainee evaluation and appraisal, should be aware of the personal and professional limitations of the trainee which could impede future professional performance. Counselor educators and supervisors have the responsibility for assisting the trainee in securing remedial assistance and screening from those trainees who are unable to provide competent services.

8. Counselor educators and supervisors should make their trainees and supervisees aware of ethical standards and legal responsibilities of the profession which they are entering and in which they are functioning.

9. Counselor educators and supervisors should have the same respect for their trainees as counselors have for their counselees. Expectations should be made clear. Allowances should be made for freedom of choice. Under no circumstances should counselor educators and supervisors attempt to sway trainees to adopt a particular theoretical belief or point of view.

10. Counselor educators and supervisors are obligated to develop clear policies regarding field placement and the roles of the trainee and field supervisor.

11. Forms of training that focus on self-understanding/growth should be voluntary unless the experience is a required part of the training program and is made known to prospective trainees prior to entering the program. When the training program requires a growth experience involving self-disclosure or other relatively intimate or personal involvement, the counselor educators and supervisors should have no administrative, supervisory or evaluative authority over the participants during the growth experience.

12. Counselor educators and supervisors are obligated to conduct training programs in keeping with the most current guidelines and/or standards of APGA, ACES and its various divisions, and state guidelines.

13. Counselor educators and supervisors have responsibility for promoting and providing opportunities for counselor educator and supervisee growth and development. They must see that staff members are adequately supervised as to the quality of their functioning.

14. Counselor educators and supervisors should not teach or supervise in any area in which they are not competent. Furthermore, counselor educators and supervisors should have adequate experience in the areas in which they are teaching or supervising.

15. Copies of all notes, records, recommendations and evaluations of supervisee and trainee performance should be made routinely available.

SUPERVISION

1. Counselor educators and supervisors should not endorse a trainee for certification, licensing or program completion if they believe that the trainee's present state of mental health would in any way interfere with the performance of counseling functions.
2. Counselor education programs should accept only those candidates who meet identified entry level requirements for admission to a program in counselor education.
3. Counselor educators should provide a realistic balance of instruction between theoretical models and practical applications.
4. Counselor educators should keep abreast of the job market and adapt programs and/or adjust number of incoming students accordingly.
5. Counselor educators and supervisors should provide practicing counselors with in-service opportunities to keep abreast of current counseling theories, practices, innovations, and issues.
6. Counselor supervisors should provide the practicing counselor with honest, periodic feedback on his or her performance.
7. Counselor educators should conduct regular follow-up studies of graduates to obtain data on the program's effectiveness and relevancy.
8. Practicum/field work sites should be carefully selected to ensure that trainees are provided satisfactory training and supervision.
9. Practicum supervisors should be provided with periodic opportunities by counselor educators to discuss current professional practices and expectations, and share ideas and mutual concerns.
10. Practicum classes should be limited in size according to ACES Standards to ensure that each student has ample opportunity for individual feedback and supervision.
11. Counselor educators should require at least minimum standards with regard to the practicum/field work experience of graduate students. Such standards should be consistent with ACES standards for preparaton in counselor education. In particular, no field work setting should be approved unless it truly replicates a potential counseling work setting.

Appendix B

The Hart Scale for Assessing Supervision

Supervision Assessment Scale
Dr. Gordon M. Hart
Developed 1979
Revised January 1981

1. Client's personality dynamics
   A. Focus on aspects of client's behavior including motivations and attitudes
   Examples: *"He is really expressing the anger inside him."*
   "How would you describe her?"
   B. Relationships and interactions with family members
   Examples: *"She takes over in the family."*
   "His mother manipulates him."
2. Case Management
   A. Referrals, treatment modes, information gathering, coordination with other agencies and supplemental assessments
   B. Conceptualizations of the management of the case
   C. What you need to know and how you will find out
   Examples: *"I feel that you owe it to your client to get all the information available from family, school, and social agencies."*
   "Do you think she needs to be referred?"
   "Have you thought about getting the family together?"
3. Treatment goals
   Examples: *"A goal would be to make him more aware of his feelings."*
   "She wants to become more assertive."
4. Counseling techniques
   A. Reference to a technique
   Example: *"How did she do on her assignment from last week?"*
   B. Prescribing a technique
   Example: *"It seems that with this client behavioral rehearsal would be appropriate."*
   C. Evaluating techniques used
   Example: *"Did you check with your client as to how she's doing on her diet?"*
5. Client-counselor relationship and interactions
   A. Statements focusing on the feelings, attitudes, and behaviors specific to the relationship and interactions between client and counselor involved

    B. Expectations in the specific relationship

        Examples: *"How have you felt in the role playing situation?"*

                "She seems resistant to your challenging her."

                "You seem to be acting condescending to him."

6. Counselor-supervisor relationship and interactions

    A. Feelings, attitudes, and behaviors specific to the present relationship and interactions between counselor and supervisor

        Examples: *"You seem angry at me."*

                "Are you becoming overly dependent on my feedback?"

                "I'm getting a feeling that you want an answer to this problem."

    B. Relationship enhancing and rapport building statements

        Example: *"I think you're doing a fine job."*

              "Are you feeling better today?"

7. Parallel process

    A. Parallels in the interactions between counselor and client and counselor and supervisor

        Example: *"You seem to be feeling helpless with your client in the sessions and now I am feeling helpless with you."*

    B. Parallels in the interactions between client and others and client and counselor

        Example: *"She gets her parents angry at her and now she has gotten you angry at her."*

    C. Other parallels such as between counselor and client and supervisor with other clients

        Example: *"I wonder why it is that you're particularly invested in this guy? That's something I like to try to figure out for myself, why it is that I particularly get into certain clients or others turn me off."*

8. Counselor's feelings, attitudes, and behavior about himself or herself

    A. Motivations, general self feelings, past behavior and general relations and interactions with persons other than the client

        Examples: *"Where is your defensiveness coming from?"*

*"Were you dependent in your relationship
with your mother?"*
*"What does that say about how you deal with
anger in your life?"*

B.   General relationship
Example: *"Do you feel that way with other clients?"*

Directions for raters:

Rate each of the numbered supervisor statements on the typescript with the number of the category on the scale that best fits
the supervisor's statement.

Explanations:

After the raters have completed the rating of the supervision
session, combine the number of times the supervisor made statements falling in categories number 1, 2, 3, and 4. Do the same for
categories 5, 6, and 7. Repeat the process for category 8. The first
cluster (categories 1, 2, 3, 4) indicates the frequency with which
the supervisor used the Skill Development model. The second cluster (categories 5, 6, 7) indicates the frequency with which the supervisor used the Integration model. The third cluster (category 8)
indicates the frequency with which the supervisor used the Personal Growth model.

References

Abels, P. A. Group supervision of students and staff. In F. W. Kaslow and Associates, *Supervision, consultation, and staff training in the helping professions.* San Francisco: Jossey-Bass, 1977.

Abroms, G. M. Supervision as metatherapy. In F. W. Kaslow and Associates, *Supervision, consultation, and staff training in the helping professions.* San Francisco: Jossey-Bass, 1977.

Ackerman, N. Selected problems in supervised analysis. *Psychiatry,* 1953, *16,* 283–290.

Ackerman, N. Some considerations for training in family therapy. In *Career Directions* (Vol. II), East Hanover, N.J.: Sandoz Pharmaceuticals, D. J. Publications, 1973.

Aiken, W. J., Smits, S. S., & Lollar, D. J. Leadership behavior and job satisfaction in state rehabilitation agencies. *Personnel Psychology,* 1972, *46,* 517–538.

Allen, J. D. Peer group supervision in family therapy. *Child Welfare,* 1976, *60,* 183–189.

Altucher, N. Constructive use of the supervisory relationship. *Journal of Counseling Psychology,* 1967, *14,* 165–170.

Anderson, R. P., & Brown, O. H. Tape recordings and counselor trainee understandings. *Journal of Counseling Psychology,* 1955, *2,* 189–194.

Anker, J. M., & Duffey, R. F. Training group therapists: A method and evaluation. *Group Psychotherapy,* 1958, *11,* 314–319.

Apostal, R. A., & Muro, J. J. Effects of group counseling on self-reports and self-recognition abilities of counselors in training. *Counselor Education and Supervision,* 1970, *10,* 56–63.

Arbuckle, D. S. The learning of counseling: Process not product. *Journal of Counseling Psychology,* 1963, *10,* 163–168.

Arbuckle, D. S. Supervision: Learning, not counseling. *Journal of Counseling Psychology,* 1965, *12,* 90–94.

Ard, B. N. Providing clinical supervision for marriage counselors: A model for supervisor and supervisee. *The Family Coordinator*, 1973, *22*, 91–97.

Arndt, H. Effective supervision in a public welfare setting. *Public Welfare*, 1973, *31*, 50–54.

Austin, L. N. An evaluation of supervision. *Social Casework*, 1956, *37*, 375–382.

Austin, L. N. Supervision in social work. *Social Work Yearbook, 1960*, 1960, 579–586.

Austin, L. N. The changing role of the supervisor. *Smith College Studies in Social Work*, 1961, *31*, 179–195.

Balsam, A., & Balsam, R. *Becoming a psychotherapist*. Boston: Little, Brown & Co., 1974.

Balsam, A., & Garber, N. Characteristics of psychotherapy supervision. *Journal of Medical Education*, 1970, *45*, 789–797.

Banikotes, P. G. Personal growth and professional training. *Counselor Education and Supervision*, 1975, *15*, 149–152.

Barnat, M. R. Student reactions to supervision: Quests for a contract. *Professional Psychology*, 1973, *4*, 17–22.

Barton, C., & Alexander, J. F. Therapist's skills as determinants of effective systems-behavioral family therapy. *International Journal of Family Counseling*, 1977, *5*, 11–20.

Bateson, G. *Mind and nature: A necessary unity*. New York: E.P. Dutton & Company, 1979.

Beck, A. T. *Cognitive therapy and the emotional disorders*. New York: International Universities Press, 1976.

Beiser, H. R. Self-listening during supervision of psychotherapy. *Archives of General Psychiatry*, 1966, *15*, 135–139.

Benedek, T. Countertransference in the training analyst. *Bulletin of the Menninger Clinic*, 1954, *18*, 12–16.

Berengarten, S. Identifying learning patterns of individual students: An exploratory study. *Social Service Review*, 1957, *31*, 407–417.

Berg, K. S., & Stone, G. L. Effects of conceptual level and supervision structure on counselor skill development. *Journal of Counseling Psychology*, 1980, *27*, 500–509.

Berger, M. M. (Ed.). *Videotape techniques in psychiatric training and treatment*. New York: Brunner/Mazel, 1970.

Bernard, J. M. Supervisor training: A discrimination model. *Counselor Education and Supervision*, 1979, *19*, 60–68.

Bernstein, B. L., & Lecomte, C. Supervisory-type feedback effects: Feedback discrepancy level, trainee psychological differentiation, and immediate responses. *Journal of Counseling Psychology*, 1979, *26*, 295–303.

Biasco, F., & Redfering, D. L. Effects of counselor supervision on group counseling: Clients' perceived outcomes. *Counselor Education and Supervision*, 1976, *15*, 216–220.

Birchler, G. R. Live supervision and instant feedback in marriage and family therapy. *Journal of Marriage and Family Counseling*, 1975, *1*, 331–342.

Birk, J. M. Effects of counseling supervision method and preference on empathic understanding. *Journal of Counseling Psychology*, 1972, *19*, 542–546.

Black, J. M. *The basics of supervisory management: Mastering the art of effective supervision*. New York: McGraw-Hill Book Company, 1975.

Blumberg, A. Supervisory behavior and interpersonal relations. *Educational Administration Quarterly*, 1968, *4*, 34–45.

Blumberg, A. A system for analyzing supervisor-teacher interaction. In A. Simon and G. Boyer (Eds.), *Mirrors for behavior change*. Philadelphia: Research for Better Schools, 1970.

Blumberg, A., & Amidon, E. Teacher perceptions of supervisor-teacher interaction. *Administrator's Notebook*, 1965, *14*, 1–8.

Bordin, E. S. *Research strategies in psychotherapy*. New York: John Wiley & Sons, 1974.

Boyd, J. D. (Ed.). *Counselor supervision: Approaches, preparation, practices*. Muncie, Ind.: Accelerated Development, 1978.

Boyd, J. D. The behavioral approach to counselor supervision. In J. D. Boyd (Ed.), *Counselor supervision: Approaches, preparation, practices*. Muncie, Ind.: Accelerated Development, 1978.

Boylston, W. H., & Tuma, J. M. Training of mental health professionals through the use of the "Bug in the ear." *American Journal of Psychiatry*, 1972, *129*, 92–95.

Brammer, L. M., & Wassmer, A. C. Supervision in counseling and psychotherapy. In D. J. Kurpius, R. D. Baker, & I. D. Thomas (Eds.), *Supervision of applied training: A comparative review*. Westport, Conn.: Greenwood Press, 1977.

Butler, E. R., & Hansen, J. C. Facilitative training: Acquisition, retention, and modes of assessment. *Journal of Counseling Psychology*, 1973, *20*, 60–65.

Campbell, D. T., & Stanley, J. C. *Experimental and quasi-experimental designs for research*. Chicago: Rand McNally, 1963.

Caplan, G. *The theory and practice of mental health consultation*. New York: Basic Books, 1970.

Carkhuff, R. R. *Helping and human relations* (Vol. I & II). New York: Holt, Rinehart & Winston, 1969.

Carkhuff, R. R. The development of systematic human resource development models. *The Counseling Psychologist*, 1972, *3*, 4–11.

Cartwright, D., & Zander, A. *Group dynamics: Research and theory*. White Plains, N.Y.: Row, Peterson and Co., 1953.

Chessick, R. D. How the resident and the supervisor disappoint each other. *American Journal of Psychotherapy*, 1971, *25*, 272–283.

Chin-Piao, C., & Appleton, W. S. The need for extensive reform in psychiatry teaching: An investigation in treatment, ideology and learning. In T. Rothmen (Ed.), *Changing patterns in psychiatric care*. New York: Crown, 1970.

Chodoff, P. Supervision of psychotherapy with videotape: Pros and cons. *American Journal of Psychiatry*, 1972, *128*, 819–823.

Clark, C. M. On the process of counseling supervision. *Counselor Education and Supervision*, 1965, *4*, 64–67.

Cleghorn, J. M., & Levin, S. Training family therapists by setting learning objectives. *American Journal of Orthopsychiatry*, 1973, *43*, 439–446.

Coché, E. Training of group therapists. In F. W. Kaslow and Associates, *Supervision, consultation, and staff training in the helping professions*. San Francisco: Jossey-Bass, 1977.

Cogan, M. *Clinical supervision*. Boston: Houghton Mifflin Company, 1972.

Cohen, R. J., & DeBetz, B. Responsive supervision of the psychiatric resident and the clinical psychology intern. *American Journal of Psychoanalysis*, 1977, *37*, 51–64.

Collins, B. E., & Guetzkaw, H. *A social psychology of group processes for decision making.* New York: John Wiley & Sons, 1964.

Colten, S. I. Supervision: Joint encounter in learning. *Journal of Education,* 1971, *3,* 7–18.

Combs, A. W., Richards, A. C., & Richards, F. *Perceptual psychology.* New York: Harper & Row, 1976.

Conant, N. *Case studies of the supervision relationship.* Unpublished doctoral dissertation, University of Nevada, Reno, 1976.

Cooper, S. Hold the hardware: The use and abuse of tapes in teaching and learning. *American Journal of Orthopsychiatry,* 1975, *45,* 573–579.

Cormier, L. S., Hackney, H., & Segrist, A. E. Three counselor training models: A comparative study. *Counselor Education and Supervision,* 1974, *14,* 95–104.

Cruser, R. W. Opinions on supervision: A chapter study. *Social Work,* 1958, *3,* 18–25.

Danish, S. J., D'Augelli, A. R., & Brock, G. W. *Helping skills verbal response system.* Unpublished manuscript, Pennsylvania State University, 1976.

Davis, K. L., & Arvey, H. H. Dual supervision: A model for counseling and supervision. *Counselor Education and Supervision,* 1978, *17,* 293–299.

DeBell, D. E. A critical digest of the literature on psychoanalytic supervision. *Journal of the American Psychoanalytic Association,* 1963, *11,* 546–574.

Delaney, D. J. A behavioral model for the supervision of counselor candidates. *Counselor Education and Supervision,* 1972, *12,* 46–50.

Delaney, D. J. Supervising counselors in preparation. In J. D. Boyd (Ed.), *Counselor supervision: Approaches, preparation, practices.* Muncie, Ind.: Accelerated Development, 1978.

Delaney, D. J., & Moore, J. C. Students' expectations of the role of practicum supervisor. *Counselor Education and Supervision,* 1966, 6, 11–17.

Delworth, U. Post-doctoral training: Is there life after internship? In C. Loganbill (Chair), *Supervision and training: Integrating theory into agency operation.* Symposium presented at the American Psychological Association, New York City, September, 1979.

Devis, D. A. Teaching and administrative functions in supervision. *Social Work,* 1965, *46,* 83–89.

Dewald, P. A. Learning problems in psychoanalytic supervision: Diagnosis and management. *Comprehensive Psychiatry,* 1969, *10,* 107–121.

Dimick, K. M., & Krause, F. H. *Practicum manual for counseling and psychotherapy* (3rd ed.). Muncie, Ind.: Accelerated Development, 1975.

Doehrman, M. J. G. Parallel processes in supervision and psychotherapy. *Bulletin of the Menninger Clinic,* 1976, *40,* 3–104.

Doyle, W. W., Jr., Foreman, M. E., & Wales, E. Effects of supervision in the training of nonprofessional crisis-intervention counselors. *Journal of Counseling Psychology,* 1977, *24,* 72–76.

D'Zmura, T. L. Teaching of psychotherapy. The function of individual supervision in the teaching of psychotherapy. *International Psychiatry Clinics,* 1964, *1,* 377–387.

Egan, G. R. Exercises in helping skills. Monterey, CA: Brooks/Cole, 1975.

Ekstein, R., & Wallerstein, R. S. The teaching and learning of psychotherapy. New York: International Universities Press, 1958.

Ekstein, R., & Wallerstein, R. S. The teaching and learning of psychotherapy (2nd ed.). New York: International Universities Press, 1972.

Emch, M. The social context of supervision. International Journal of Psychoanalysis, 1955, 36, 298–306.

Ferber, A. Follow the paths with heart. International Journal of Psychiatry, 1972, 10, 6–22.

Fitch, J., Malley, P. B., & Scott, J. A. (co-producers). Simulation vignettes for training counselor supervisors. Pittsburgh: University of Pittsburgh, Department of Counselor Education, 1975. (Videotape)

Fleckles, C. S. The making of a psychiatrist: The resident's view of the process of his professional development. American Journal of Psychiatry, 1972, 128, 101–105.

Fleming, J. The role of supervision in psychiatric training. Bulletin of the Menninger Clinic, 1953, 17, 157–169.

Fleming, J., & Benedek, T. F. Supervision: A method of teaching psychoanalysis. Psychoanalytic Quarterly, 1964, 33, 71–96.

Fleming, J., & Benedek, T. F. Psychoanalytic supervision: A method of clinical teaching. New York: Grune & Stratton, 1966.

French, J. R. P., & Raven, B. The bases of social power. In D. Cartwright and A. Zander (Eds.), Group dynamics. Evanston, Ill.: Row and Peterson, 1960.

Gale, M. S. Resident perception of psychotherapy supervision. Comprehensive Psychiatry, 1976, 17, 191–194.

Gans, R. W. Group co-therapists and the therapeutic condition. International Journal of Group Psychotherapy, 1962, 12, 82–88.

Gaoni, B., & Neumann, M. Supervision from the point of view of the supervisee. American Journal of Psychotherapy, 1974, 24, 108–114.

Gardner, G. E. Problems of supervision and training in clinical psychology. The supervision of psychotherapy. American Journal of Orthopsychiatry, 1953, 23, 293–300.

Gazda, G. M. Group counseling: A developmental approach. Boston: Allyn and Bacon, 1971.

Gelso, C. J. Research in counseling: Methodological and professional issues. Counseling Psychologist, 1979, 8, 7–36.

Gitelson, M. Problems of psychoanalytic training. Psychoanalytic Quarterly, 1948, 17, 198–211.

Goin, M. K., & Kline, F. M. Supervision observed. Journal of Nervous and Mental Diseases, 1974, 158, 208–213.

Goldfarb, N. Effects of supervisory style on counselor effectiveness and facilitative responding. Journal of Counseling Psychology, 1978, 25, 454–460.

Goldhammer, R. Clinical supervision: Special methods for the supervision of teachers. New York: Holt, Rinehart & Winston, 1969.

Goldman, L. A revolution in counseling research. Journal of Counseling Psychology, 1976, 23, 543–552.

Gormally, J. A behavioral analysis of structured skills training. Journal of Counseling Psychology, 1975, 22, 458–460.

Grossman, W. K., & Karmol, E. Group psychotherapy supervision and its effect on resident training. *American Journal of Psychotherapy*, 1973, *130*, 920–921.

Grotjahn, M. Problems and techniques of supervision. *Psychiatry*, 1955, *18*, 9–15.

Guldner, C. Family therapy for the trainee in family therapy. *Journal of Marriage and Family Counseling*, 1978, *4*, 127–132.

Gurk, M. D., & Wicas, E. D. Generic models of counseling supervision: Counseling/instruction dichotomy and consultation metamodel. *The Personnel and Guidance Journal*, 1979, 57, 402–407.

Gysbers, N. C., & Johnston, J. A. Expectations of a practicum supervisor's role. *Counselor Education and Supervision*, 1965, *4*, 68–74.

Hackney, H., & Cormier, L. S. *Counseling strategies and objectives* (2nd ed.). Englewood Cliffs, N.J.: Prentice-Hall, 1979.

Hackney, H., & Nye, S. *Counseling strategies and objectives*. Englewood Cliffs, N.J.: Prentice-Hall, 1973.

Haley, J. *Strategies of psychotherapy*. New York: Grune & Stratton, 1963.

Haley, J. Fourteen ways to fail as a teacher of family therapy. *Family Therapy*, 1974, *1*, 1–8.

Haley, J. Why a mental health clinic should avoid family therapy. *Journal of Marriage and Family Counseling*, 1975, *1*, 3–12.

Haley, J. Problems in training therapists. In J. Haley, *Problem-solving therapy*. San Francisco: Jossey-Bass, 1976.

Hamachek, J. N. *Effects of individual supervision on selected affective and cognitive characteristics of counselors-in-training: A pilot study*. Unpublished doctoral dissertation, Michigan State University, 1971.

Hamatz, M. G. Two-channel recording in the supervision of psychotherapy. *Professional Psychology*, 1975, 6, 478–480.

Hanlan, A. Changing functions and structures. In F. W. Kaslow and Associates, *Issues in human services: A sourcebook for supervision and staff development*. San Francisco: Jossey-Bass, 1972.

Hansen, J. C. Trainees' expectations of supervision in the counseling practicum. *Counselor Education and Supervision*, 1965, *2*, 75–80.

Hansen, J. C., & Warner, R. W. Review of research on practicum supervision. *Counselor Education and Supervision*, 1971, *10*, 261–272.

Hansen, J. C., Pound, R., & Petro, C. Review of research on practicum supervision. *Counselor Education and Supervision*, 1976, *16*, 107–116.

Hansen, J. C., Stevic, R. R., & Warner, R. W. *Counseling theory and process*. Boston: Allyn and Bacon, 1972.

Hare-Mustin, R. T. Live supervision in psychotherapy. *Voices*, 1976, *12*, 21–24.

Hare, R. T., & Frankena, S. Peer group supervision. *American Journal of Orthopsychiatry*, 1972, *42*, 527–529.

Hart, G. M. (Producer). *Impasses between supervisors and supervisees*. Philadelphia: Temple University, Department of Counseling Psychology, 1974. (Videotape)

Hart, G. M. (Producer). *Styles of supervision I*. Philadelphia: Temple University, Department of Counseling Psychology, 1976. (Videotape) (a)

Hart, G. M. (Producer). *Styles of supervision II*. Philadelphia: Temple

University, Department of Counseling Psychology, 1976. (Videotape) (b)

Hart, G. M. (Producer). *Styles of supervision III*. Philadelphia: Temple University, Department of Counseling Psychology, 1976. (Videotape) (c)

Hart, G. M. (Producer). *Critical moments in supervision I*. Philadelphia: Temple University, Department of Counseling Psychology, 1976. (Videotape) (d)

Hart, G. M. (Producer). *Critical moments in supervision II*. Philadelphia: Temple University, Department of Counseling Psychology, 1976. (Videotape) (e)

Hart, G. M. Models of supervision in the helping professions. In H. A. Liddle and G. M. Hart (Co-chairs), *The many faces of supervision: A videotape demonstration*. Presentation at the annual meeting of the American Personnel and Guidance Association, Washington, D.C., March 1978. (a)

Hart, G. M. Continuing professional development: The outlook for counselor educators and supervisors. *Counselor Education and Supervision*, 1978, *18*, 116–125. (b)

Hart, G. M. *Striving for excellence: The preservice and inservice training of counselors*. Ann Arbor, MI.: ERIC/CAPS, 1979. (Monograph) (a)

Hart, G. M. *Development of an instrument to determine models of supervision*. Unpublished manuscript, Temple University, Department of Counseling Psychology, 1979. (b)

Hart, G. M., & Liddle, H. A. (Co-producers). *The process of group supervision*. Philadelphia: Temple University, Department of Counseling Psychology, 1976. (Videotape)

Hart, G. M., Maslin, A., Liberi, W. P., & Wondolowski, M. *Styles of supervision I: Instructor manual*. Philadelphia: Temple University, Department of Counseling Psychology, 1976. (a)

Hart, G. M., Maslin, A., Liberi, W. P., & Wondolowski, M. *Styles of supervision II: Instructor manual*. Philadelphia: Temple University, Department of Counseling Psychology, 1976. (b)

Hart, G. M., Maslin, A., Liberi, W. P., & Wondolowski, M. *Styles of supervision III: Instructor manual*. Philadelphia: Temple University, Department of Counseling Psychology, 1976. (c)

Hart, G. M., Maslin, A., Liberi, W. P., & Wondolowski, M. *Critical moments in supervision I: Instructor manual*. Philadelphia: Temple University, Department of Counseling Psychology, 1976. (d)

Hart, G. M., Maslin, A., Liberi, W. P., & Wondolowski, M. *Critical moments in supervision II: Instructor manual*. Philadelphia: Temple University, Department of Counseling Psychology, 1976. (e)

Heck, E. J. Research information on counseling laboratory students. Paper presented at the annual meeting of the American Personnel and Guidance Association, Chicago, April, 1976.

Heckel, W. H., Malley, P. B., Scott, J. A., & Spice, G. C. (Co-producers). *Triadic supervision*. Pittsburgh: University of Pittsburgh, Department of Counselor Education, 1975. (Videotape)

Hendrickson, D. E., & Krause, F. H. (Eds.). *Counseling and psychotherapy: Training and supervision*. Columbus, Ohio: Merrill, 1972.

Hester, L. R., Weitz, L. J., Anchor, K. N., & Roback, H. B. Supervisor attraction as a function of supervisor skillfulness and supervisees' perceived similarity. *Journal of Counseling Psychology*, 1976, *23*, 254–258.

Hewer, V. An aid to supervision in practicum. *Journal of Counseling Psychology*, 1974, *21*, 66–70.

Hogan, R. A. Issues and approaches in supervision. *Psychotherapy: Theory, research and practice*, 1964, *1*, 139–141.

Howe, L. W., & Howe, M. M. *Personalizing education: Values clarification and beyond*. New York: Hart, 1975.

Hutt, M. L. Problems of supervision and training in clinical psychology. Discussion. *American Journal of Orthopsychiatry*, 1953, *23*, 328–331.

Ivey, A. E. *Microcounseling: Innovations in interviewing training* (2nd ed.). Springfield, Ill.: Charles C. Thomas, 1978.

Jourard, S. M. *The transparent self*. (Rev. ed.). New York: Van Nostrand Reinhold, 1971.

Kadis, A., & Markowitz, M. Short-term analytic treatment of married couples in a group by a therapist couple. In C. Sager and H. Kaplan (Eds.), *Progress in group and family therapy*. New York: Brunner/Mazel, 1972.

Kadushin, A. Games people play in supervision. *Social Work*, 1968, *13*, 23–32.

Kadushin, A. *Supervisor-supervisee: A questionnaire study*. Unpublished manuscript, University of Wisconsin, School of Social Work, 1973.

Kadushin, A. Supervisor-supervisee: A survey. *Social Work*, 1974, *19*, 288–298.

Kadushin, A. *Supervision in social work*. New York: Columbia University Press, 1976.

Kagan, N. Influencing human interaction—eleven years with IPR. *Canadian Counselor*, 1975, *9*, 74–97.

Kagan, N., & Krathwohl, D. R. *Studies in human interaction: Interpersonal process recall stimulated by videotape*. East Lansing, MI.: Educational Publishing Services, 1967.

Kagan, N., Krathwohl, D. R., & Miller, R. Stimulated recall in therapy using videotape: A case study. *Journal of Counseling Psychology*, 1963, *10*, 237–243.

Kagan, N., & Schauble, P. G. Affect simulation in interpersonal recall. *Journal of Counseling Psychology*, 1969, *16*, 309–313.

Kagan, N., Schauble, P. G., Resnikoff, A., Danish, S. J., & Krathwohl, D. R. Interpersonal process recall. *Journal of Nervous and Mental Disease*, 1969, *148*, 365–374.

Kagan, N., & Werner, A. Supervision in psychiatric education. In D. J. Kurpius, R. D. Baker, & I. D. Thomas (Eds.), *Supervison of applied training: A comparative review*. Westport, Conn.: Greenwood Press, 1977.

Kaplowitz, D. Teaching empathic responsiveness in the supervisory process of psychotherapy. *American Journal of Psychotherapy*, 1967, *21*, 774–781.

Kaslow, F. W., & Associates. Issues in human services: A sourcebook for supervision and staff development. San Francisco: Jossey-Bass, 1972.

Kaslow, F. W. and Associates. *Supervision, consultation, and staff training in the helping professions.* San Francisco: Jossey-Bass, 1977.

Kaslow, F. W. Training of marital and family therapists. In F. W. Kaslow and Associates, *Supervision, consultation, and staff training in the helping professions.* San Francisco: Jossey-Bass, 1977.

Kaslow, F. W. Community mental health centers. In F. W. Kaslow and Associates, *Supervision, consultation, and staff training in the helping professions.* San Francisco: Jossey-Bass, 1977.

Kell, B. L., & Mueller, W. J. *Impact and change: A study of counseling relationships.* Englewood Cliffs, N.J.: Prentice-Hall, 1966.

Kendall, D. A. *A comparison of two approaches to a counseling practicum.* Unpublished doctoral dissertation, University of Pittsburgh, 1972.

Kermish, J., & Kushin, F. Why high turnover? Social work staff losses in a county welfare agency. *Public Welfare,* 1969, *27,* 134–137.

Kimberlin, C., & Friesen, D. Effects of client ambivalence, trainee conceptual level, and empathy training conditions on empathic responding. *Journal of Counseling Psychology,* 1977, *24,* 354–358.

Kirchner, K. R. *Expectations about individual counseling supervision.* Unpublished doctoral dissertation, University of Missouri, 1974.

Kledarias, C. G. *A study of the role conflict in supervision.* Unpublished doctoral dissertation, Catholic University of America, 1971.

Krumboltz, J. D. Changing the behavior of behavior changers. *Counselor Education and Supervision,* 1967, *6,* 222–229.

Kurpius, D. J., & Baker, R. D. The supervisory process: Analysis and synthesis. In D. J. Kurpius, R. D. Baker, & I. D. Thomas (Eds.), *Supervision of applied training: A comparative review.* Westport, Conn.: Greenwood Press, 1977.

Kurpius, D. J., Baker, R. D., & Thomas, I. D. (Eds.). *Supervision of applied training: A comparative review.* Westport, Conn.: Greenwood Press, 1977.

Kurpius, D. J., & Robinson, S. E. An overview of consultation. *Personnel and Guidance Journal,* 1978, *56,* 321–323.

Kurtz, R. M., & Kaplan, M. L. Resident attitude development and the ideological commitment of the staff of psychiatric training institutions. *Journal of Medical Education,* 1968, *15,* 516–525.

Kutzik, A. J. Class and ethnic factors. In F. W. Kaslow and Associates, *Issues in human services: A sourcebook for supervision and staff development.* San Francisco: Jossey-Bass, 1972.

Kutzik, A. J. The medical field. In F. W. Kaslow and Associates, *Supervision, consultation, and staff training in the helping professions.* San Francisco: Jossey-Bass, 1977.

Lakin, M. *Interpersonal encounter: Theory and practice in sensitivity training.* New York: McGraw-Hill, 1972.

Lambert, M. J. Supervisory and counseling process: A comparative study. *Counselor Education and Supervision,* 1974, *14,* 54–60.

Lear, M., & Hart, G. M. *Peer group supervision in a community agency.* Unpublished manuscript, Temple University, Department of Counseling Psychology, 1980.

Leary, T. *Interpersonal diagnosis of personality.* New York: Ronald Press, 1957.

Leddick, G. R., & Bernard, J. M. The history of supervision: A critical review. *Counselor Education and Supervision*, 1980, *19*, 186–196.

Levin, E. M., & Kurtz, R. R. Structured and nonstructured human relations training. *Journal of Counseling Psychology*, 1974, *21*, 526–531.

Liberi, W. P. *The effect of group supervision on self-concept, interpersonal orientation, and counseling skills.* Unpublished doctoral dissertation, Temple University, 1978.

Liddle, H. A. The emotional and political hazards of teaching and learning family therapy. *Family Therapy*, 1978, 5, 1–12.

Liddle, H. A. Training contextual therapists: Steps toward an integrative model of training and supervision. In P. Sholevar (Ed.), *Marriage, marital, and divorce therapy.* New York: Springer, 1979.

Liddle, H. A., & Halpin, R. J. Family therapy training and supervision literature: A comparative review. *Journal of Marriage and Family Counseling*, 1978, *4*, 77–98.

Liddle, H. A., & Smith, J. P. *Report of the Community Counseling Clinic-1976–77.* Unpublished manuscript, Temple University, Department of Counseling Psychology, 1977.

Liddle, H. A., & Smith, J. P. *Report of the Community Counseling Clinic 1977–78.* Unpublished manuscript, Temple University, Department of Counseling Psychology, 1978.

Liddle, H. A., Tannenbaum, A., & Maloy, C. *Effects of live supervision: The trainee's perspective.* Paper presented at the annual meeting of the American Orthopsychiatric Association, Montreal, April, 1980.

Lister, J. L. Counselor experiencing: Its implications for supervision. *Counselor Education and Supervision*, 1966, 5, 55–60. (a)

Lister, J. L. Supervised counseling experiences: Some comments. *Counselor Education and Supervision*, 1966, 6, 69–72. (b)

Littrell, J. M. Concerns of beginning counselor trainees. *Counselor Education and Supervision*, 1978, *18*, 29–35.

Littrell, J. M., Lee-Borden, N., & Lorenz, J. A developmental framework for counseling supervision. *Counselor Education and Supervision*, 1979, *19*, 129–136.

Loganbill, C. A developmental approach to supervision: Specific training techniques. In C. Loganbill (Chair), *Supervision and training: Integrating theory into agency operation.* Symposium presented at the annual meeting of the American Psychological Association, New York City, September, 1979.

Mahon, B. R., & Altmann, H. A. Skill training: Cautions and recommendations. *Counselor Education and Supervision*, 1977, *17*, 42–50.

Mahoney, M. J. *Cognition and behavior modification.* Cambridge, Mass.: Ballinger, 1974.

Markey, M. J., Frederickson, R. H., Johnson, R. W., & Julius, M. A. Influence of playback technique on counselor performance. *Counselor Education and Supervision*, 1970, 9, 178–182.

Matarazzo, R. G. Research on the teaching and learning of psychotherapy skills. In S. L. Garfield and A. E. Bergin (Eds.), *Handbook of psychotherapy and behavior change: An empirical analysis* (2nd ed.). New York: John Wiley & Sons, 1978.

Mathews, W. M., & Wineman, D. Problems of supervision and training in clinical psychology. The supervision of clinical diagnostic work. *Amer-*

ican Journal of Orthopsychiatry, 1953, *23,* 293–300.

McElhose, R. T. *Supervisor-supervisee complimentarity and relational distance as related to supervisor experience level.* Unpublished doctoral dissertation, Michigan State University, 1973.

McGee, T. F. Supervision in group psychotherapy: A comparison of four approaches. *International Journal of Group Psychotherapy,* 1968, *18,* 165–176.

McGee, T. F. The triadic approach to supervision in group psychotherapy. *International Journal of Group Psychotherapy,* 1974, *24,* 471–476.

McGee, T. F., & Schuman, B. N. The nature of the co-therapy relationship. *International Journal of Group Psychotherapy,* 1970, *20,* 25–36.

McKinnon, D. W. Group counseling with student counselors. *Counselor Education and Supervision,* 1969, *8,* 195–200.

McLennan, B. W. Co-therapy. *International Journal of Group Psychotherapy,* 1965, *5,* 154–166.

Melchiode, G. A. Psychoanalytically oriented individual therapy. In F. W. Kaslow and Associates, *Supervision, consultation, and staff training in the helping professions.* San Francisco: Jossey-Bass, 1977.

Meltzer, R. School and agency cooperation in using videotape in social work education. *Journal of Education for Social Work,* 1977, *13,* 90–95.

Mezzano, J. A note on dogmatism and counselor effectiveness. *Counselor Education and Supervision,* 1969, *9,* 64–65.

Miller, C. D., & Oetting, E. R. Students react to supervision. *Counselor Education and Supervision,* 1966, *6,* 73–74.

Minuchin, S. *Families and family therapy.* Cambridge, Mass.: Harvard University Press, 1974.

Montalvo, B. Aspects of live supervision. *Family Process,* 1973, *12,* 343–359.

Moore, M. The client's voice in supervision. *Voices,* 1969, *5,* 76–78.

Morgan, S. M. *The relationship between congruent student and supervisor expectations, student performance, and student satisfaction in counseling practica.* Unpublished doctoral dissertation, University of Tennessee, 1976.

Mosher, R. L., & Purpel, D. E. *Supervision: The reluctant profession.* Boston: Houghton Mifflin, 1972.

Mueller, W. J., & Kell, B. L. *Coping with conflict: Supervising counselors and psychotherapists.* New York: Appleton-Century-Crofts, 1972.

Muslin, H. L., Burstein, A. G., Gedo, J. E., & Sadow, L. Research on the supervisory process: I. Supervisors' appraisal of the interview data. *Archives of General Psychiatry,* 1967, *16,* 427–431.

Napier, R. E. *Counselor development: Longitudinal study of the association between trainee effectiveness and supervisory relationship.* Unpublished doctoral dissertation, University of Ottawa, 1979.

Nash, V. C. *The clinical supervision of psychotherapy.* Unpublished doctoral dissertation, Yale University, 1975.

Nelson, G. Psychotherapy supervision from the trainee's point of view: A survey of preferences. *Professional Psychology,* 1978, *9,* 539–550.

Newton, R. *Supervisor expectations and behavior: Effects of consistent-inconsistent supervisory pairings on supervisee satisfaction with supervision, perceptions of supervisory relationships and rated counselor competency.* Unpublished doctoral dissertation, University of Missouri, 1976.

O'Connor, C. T. Group influences on the choice of a psychiatric viewpoint. *Archives of General Psychiatry*, 1965, *13*, 429–431.

Ohlsen, M. M. *Group Counseling* (2nd ed.). New York: Holt, Rinehart & Winston, 1977.

Olmstead, J., & Christensen, H. E. *Effects of agency work contexts: An intensive field study* (Research Report No. 2). Washington, D. C.: Department of Health, Education, and Welfare, 1973.

Olyan, S. D. *An exploratory study of supervision in Jewish community centers as compared to other welfare settings.* Unpublished doctoral dissertation, University of Pittsburgh, 1972.

Oratio, A. R. *Supervision in speech pathology: A handbook for supervisors and clinicians.* Baltimore: University Park Press, 1977.

Papp, P. The family who had all the answers. In P. Papp (Ed.), *Family therapy: Full length case studies.* New York: Gardner Press, 1977.

Patterson, C. H. Supervising students in the counseling practicum. *Journal of Counseling Psychology*, 1964, *11*, 47–53.

Payne, P. A., & Gralinski, D. M. Effects of supervisor style and empathy upon counselor learning. *Journal of Counseling Psychology*, 1968, *15*, 517–521.

Payne, P. A., Weiss, S. D., & Kapp, R. A. Didactic, experiential, and modeling factors in the learning of empathy. *Journal of Counseling Psychology*, 1972, *19*, 425–429.

Payne, P. A., Winter, D. E., & Bell, G. E. Effects of supervisor style on the learning of empathy in a supervision analogue. *Counselor Education and Supervision*, 1972, *11*, 262–269.

Peter, L. F., & Hull, R. *The Peter principle.* New York: Morrow, 1969.

Pettes, D. E. *Supervision in social work: A method of student training and staff development.* London: Allen & Unwin, 1967.

Pfeiffer, J. W., Heslin, R., & Jones, J. E. *Instrumentation in human relations training* (2nd ed.). La Jolla, CA: University Associates, 1973.

Pfeiffer, J. W., & Jones, J. E. *A handbook of structured experiences for human relations training.* Iowa City: University Associates, 1969.

Pierce, R. M., & Schauble, P. G. Graduate training of facilitative counselors: The effects of individual supervision. *Journal of Counseling Psychology*, 1970, *17*, 210–215.

Pierce, R. M., & Schauble, P. G. Follow-up study of the effects of individual supervision in graduate school training. *Journal of Counseling Psychology*, 1971, *18*, 186–187. (a)

Pierce, R. M., & Schauble, P. G. Toward the development of facilitative counselors: The effects of practicum instruction and individual supervision. *Counselor Education and Supervision*, 1971, *11*, 83–89. (b)

Poling, E. G. Videotape recordings in counseling practicum: I—Environmental considerations. *Counselor Education and Supervision*, 1968, *7*, 348–356. (a)

Poling, E. G. Videotape recordings in counseling practicum: II—Critique considerations. *Counselor Education and Supervision*, 1968, *8*, 33–38. (b)

Rapoport, L. The use of supervision as a tool in professional development. *British Journal of Psychiatric Social Work*, 1954, *2*, 66–74.

Reavis, C. A. *Teacher improvement through clinical supervision.* Bloomington, Ind.: Phi Delta Kappa, 1978.

Resnikoff, A., Kagan, N., & Schauble, P. G. Acceleration of psychotherapy through stimulated videotape recall. *American Journal of Psychotherapy*, 1970, *24*, 102–111.

Rhim, B. C. The use of videotapes in social work agencies. *Social Casework*, 1976, *57*, 644–650.

Rogers, C. R. *Client-centered therapy*. Boston: Houghton Mifflin, 1951.

Rogers, C. R. Training individuals to engage in the therapeutic process. In C. R. Strother (Ed.), *Psychology and mental health*. Washington, D.C.: American Psychological Association, 1957.

Rosenbaum, M. Problems in supervision of psychiatric residents in psychotherapy. *American Medical Association Archives of Neurology and Psychiatry*, 1953, *69*, 43–48.

Rosenberg, L. M., Rubin, S. S., & Finzi, H. Participant-supervision in the teaching of psychotherapy. *American Journal of Psychotherapy*, 1968, *22*, 280–295.

Rosenthal, N. R. A prescriptive approach for counselor training. *Journal of Counseling Psychology*, 1977, *24*, 231–237.

Rubinstein, D. Family therapy. In H. Hoffman (Ed.). *Teaching of psychotherapy: International psychiatric clinics* (Vol. I). Boston: Little, Brown & Co., 1964.

Schauble, P. G. *The acceleration of client progress in counseling and psychotherapy through interpersonal process recall (IPR)*. Unpublished doctoral dissertation, Michigan State University, 1970.

Schiff, S. B., & Reivich, R. Use of television as aid to psychotherapy supervision. *Archives of General Psychiatry*, 1964, *10*, 84–88.

Schlessinger, N. Supervision of psychotherapy. *Archives of General Psychiatry*, 1966, *15*, 129–134.

Schowalter, J. E., & Pruett, K. The supervision process for individual child psychotherapy. *Journal of the American Academy of Child Psychiatry*, 1975, *14*, 708–718.

Schuster, D. B., & Freeman, E. N. Supervision of the resident's initial interview. *Archives of General Psychiatry*, 1970, *23*, 516–523.

Schuster, D. B., Sandt, J. J., & Thaler, O. F. *Clinical supervision of the psychiatric resident*. New York: Brunner/Mazel, 1972.

Schwartz, E. E., & Sample, W. C. *The midway office: An experiment in the organization of work groups*. New York: National Association of Social Workers, 1972.

Scott, R. W. Professional employees in a bureaucratic structure. In A. Etzioni, (Ed.), *The semiprofessions and their organization*. New York: Free Press, 1969.

Searles, H. F. The informational value of the supervisor's emotional experiences. *Psychiatry*, 1955, *18*, 135–146.

Seligman, L. The relationship of facilitative functioning to effective peer supervision. *Counselor Education and Supervision*, 1978, *17*, 254–261.

Semrad, E. J., & Van Buskirk, D. (Eds.). *Teaching psychotherapy of psychotic patients*. New York: Grune & Stratton, 1969.

Sharaf, M. R., & Levinson, D. J. Patterns of ideology and professional role definition among psychiatric residents. In M. Greenblatt, D. Levinson, & R. Williams (Eds.), *The patient and the mental hospital*. Glencoe, Ill.: Free Press, 1957.

Silverman, M. S., & Quinn, P. F. Co-counseling supervision in practicum. *Counselor Education and Supervision*, 1974, *13*, 256–260.

Simon, A., & Boyer, G. (Eds.). *Mirrors for behavior change.* Philadelphia: Research for Better Schools, 1970.

Simon, S. B., Howe, L. W., & Kirschenbaum, H. *Values clarification: A handbook of practical strategies for teachers and students.* New York: Hart, 1972.

Smith, J. P. *Supervisor behavior and supervisor expectations.* Unpublished doctoral dissertation, University of Missouri, 1975.

Spice, C. G., & Spice, W. H. A triadic method of supervision in the training of counselors and counseling supervisors. *Counselor Education and Supervision*, 1976, *15*, 251–258.

Spiegel, P., & Grunebaum, H. Training versus treating the psychiatric resident. *American Journal of Psychotherapy*, 1977, *31*, 618–625.

Stein, S. P., Karasu, T. B., Charles, E. S., & Buckley, P. J. Supervision of the initial interview. *Archives of General Psychiatry*, 1975, *32*, 265–268.

Stoller, F. H. Use of videotape (focused feedback) in group counseling and group therapy. In G. Gazda (Ed.), *Innovations to group psychotherapy.* Springfield, Ill.: Charles C Thomas, 1968.

Stone, G. L. Effects of experience on supervisor planning. *Journal of Counseling Psychology*, 1980, *27*, 84–88.

Strauss, A. L. *Psychiatric ideologies and institutions.* New York: Free Press, 1964.

Sullivan, H. S. *Conceptions of modern psychiatry* (2nd ed.). New York: W. W. Norton & Company, 1953.

Sullivan, H. S. *Clinical studies in psychiatry.* New York: W. W. Norton & Company, 1956.

Tarachow, S. *An introduction to psychotherapy.* New York: International Universities Press, 1963.

Tentoni, S. C., & Robb, G. P. Improving the counseling practicum through immediate radio feedback. *College Student Journal*, 1977, *12*, 279–283.

Thoresen, C. E. Counseling research: What I can't help thinking. *The Counseling Psychologist*, 1979, *8*, 56–61.

Tinsley, H. E. A., & Tinsley, D. J. Relationship between scores on the Omnibus Personality Inventory and counselor trainee effectiveness. *Journal of Counseling Psychology*, 1977, *24*, 522–526.

Todd, W. E., & Pine, I. Peer supervision of individual psychotherapy. *American Journal of Psychiatry*, 1968, *125*, 780–784.

Tomm, K. M., & Wright, L. M. Training in family therapy: Perceptual, conceptual and executive skills. *Family Process*, 1979, *18*, 227–250.

Toukmanian, S. G., & Rennie, D. L. Microcounseling versus human relations training: Relative effectiveness with undergraduate trainees. *Journal of Counseling Psychology*, 1975, *22*, 345–352.

Truax, C. B., Carkhuff, R. R., & Douds, J. Toward an integration of didactic and experiential approaches to training in counseling and psychotherapy. *Journal of Counseling Psychology*, 1964, *11*, 240–247.

Tucker, B. Z., Hart, G. M., & Liddle, H. A. Supervision in family therapy: A developmental perspective. *Journal of Marriage and Family Counseling*, 1976, *2*, 260–276.

Tucker, B. Z., & Liddle, H. A. Intra- and interpersonal processes in the group supervision of family therapists. *Family Therapy*, 1978, *5*, 13–27.

Van Atta, R. E. Co-therapy as a supervisory process. *Psychotherapy: Theory, research, and practice*, 1969, 6, 137–139.

Vargus, I. D. Supervision in social work. In D. J. Kurpius, R. D. Baker, & I. D. Thomas (Eds.), *Supervision of applied training: A comparative review*. Westport, Conn.: Greenwood Press, 1977.

Wagner, C. A., & Smith, J. P. Peer supervision: Toward more effective training. *Counselor Education and Supervision*, 1979, 18, 288–293.

Walz, G. R., & Johnston, J. A. Counselors look at themselves on videotape. *Journal of Counseling Psychology*, 1963, 10, 232–236.

Walz, G. R., & Roeber, E. C. Supervisors' reactions to a counseling interview. *Counselor Education and Supervision*, 1962, 1, 2–7.

Ward, G. R., Kagan, N., & Krathwohl, D. R. An attempt to measure and facilitate counselor effectiveness. *Counselor Education and Supervision*, 1972, 11, 179–186.

Warnath, C. F. Relationship and growth theories and agency counseling. *Counselor Education and Supervision*, 1977, 17, 84–91.

Wasserman, H. Early careers of professional social workers in a public child welfare agency. *Social Work*, 1970, 15, 93–101.

Watson, D. C., & Tharp, R. G. *Self-directed behavior: Self-modification for personal adjustment* (2nd ed.). Monterey, CA: Brooks/Cole, 1977.

Watson, K. W. Differential supervision. *Social Work*, 1973, 18, 80–88.

Whitaker, C. Comment. Live supervision in psychotherapy. *Voices*, 1976, 12, 24–25.

Wilbur, M. P. *The association among nonverbal stimuli, supervisory strategies, and satisfaction ratings in counselor-trainee supervision*. Unpublished doctoral dissertation, Western Michigan University, 1975.

Wilbur, M. P., & Wilbur, J. R. Counselor educator nonverbal behavior in the supervision process. *Counselor Education and Supervision*, 1979, 19, 101–109.

Wiles, K., & Lovell, J. T. *Supervision for better schools*. Englewood Cliffs, N.J.: Prentice-Hall, 1975.

Williamson, M. *Supervision: New patterns and processes*. New York: Association Press, 1961.

Windholz, E. The theory of supervision in psychoanalytic education. *International Journal of Psychoanalysis*, 1970, 51, 393–406.

Winstead, D. K., Bonowitz, J. S., Gale, M. S., & Evans, J. W. Resident peer supervision of psychotherapy. *American Journal of Psychiatry*, 1974, 131, 318–321.

Wolberg, L. R. Supervision of the psychotherapeutic process. *American Journal of Psychotherapy*, 1951, 5, 147–171.

Worthington, E. L., Jr., & Roehlke, H. J. Effective supervision as perceived by beginning counselors-in-training. *Journal of Counseling Psychology*, 1979, 26, 64–73.

Yalom, I. D. *The theory and practice of group psychotherapy* (2nd ed.). New York: Basic Books, 1975.

Yenawine, G., & Arbuckle, D. S. Study of the use of videotape and audiotape as techniques in counselor education. *Journal of Counseling Psychology*, 1971, 18, 1–6.

Index